THE HEARING IMPAIRED CHILD
AND SCHOOL

HUMAN HORIZONS SERIES

The Hearing Impaired Child and School

Ivan Tucker and Con Powell

A CONDOR BOOK
Souvenir Press E&A Ltd

First published 1991 by Souvenir Press (Educational & Academic) Ltd, 43 Great Russell Street, London WC1B 3PA and simultaneously in Canada.

ISBN 0 285 650785 hardback
ISBN 0 285 650793 paperback

Printed and bound in Great Britain
by WBC Ltd., Bridgend, Mid Glamorgan.

Contents

Introduction   vii

1   Understanding Hearing Impairment   1

2   Understanding Amplification   24

3   Communication Approaches Used in the Education of Hearing Impaired Children   57

4   The Range of Educational Options for Hearing Impaired Children   84

5   Educational Placement   123

6   Hearing Impaired Children and the National Curriculum   142

7   Listening in Ordinary Classrooms   155

8   The Child with Handicaps Additional to Deafness   168

Appendix: Useful Addresses   179

Index   185

Introduction

The Hearing Impaired Child and the Family, published in 1981, offered support and some guidance to the families of young hearing impaired children. This was presented as they tried to come to terms with deafness, what it means, the diagnosis and early treatment of their child and above all how they might help him or her to develop. It was intended that the book should be easy to read and reviewers indicate some success in that aim; the work is now in its second edition, greatly updated in 1988.

The publishers always thought that it should be followed by a book, again primarily but not solely for parents, on hearing impaired children in school, outlining the range of possibilities that are available in some areas and which we believe should be available everywhere.

There have been massive changes in the climate in which education is taking place and there have been substantial changes in the legislative framework, all of which we wish to comment on. We hope that this will not be too dull for you to read, we are quite sure that it is essential that you do read information that outlines the responsibilities of local education authorities and gives you an idea of what your rights are as a parent of a hearing impaired child.

We hope that there will be much else in the book to interest and inform you. Included is information about the available range of educational options—the mainstream class, the resource base, the partially hearing unit, the day special and the residential special school, etc.—and comment on the advantages and disadvantages of each form of provision. Where appropriate, material is also included on the child with difficulties additional to deafness.

Stress is placed on the requirements for in-service training and support of mainstream teachers who increasingly have hearing impaired children in their classes. As you might expect, we put great emphasis on the problems of effective use of hearing aids in noisy mainstream environments where so many hearing impaired children are currently placed, and suggest some ways of maximising the benefits of hearing aids for the child so placed.

As in *The Hearing Impaired Child and the Family*, we stress ways in which parents and teachers can co-operate to the benefit of the child. We try, as gently as possible, to persuade parents that after the tremendous effort of the pre-school years they cannot 'retire' from active involvement. The child still needs their input and will still benefit from co-operation with professionals as he or she develops towards being an educated, fully rounded personality.

1. Understanding Hearing Impairment

In this book our major aim will be to explore the educational management of children in a variety of school settings but prior to this we need to explain for many teachers the 'whys' and 'wherefores' of deafness, since it is possible that they, like the population at large, will have preconceived and possibly inaccurate ideas about deafness, what causes it, where the damage is, and whether there is a cure for it.

STRUCTURE AND MECHANISM OF THE EAR

In order to understand deafness we need to consider at least in a little detail the anatomy and physiology of the hearing mechanism, concentrating on the parts of the ear to the point where sound stimuli are transformed into electrical energy in the nervous system. Some consideration is also given to the neural pathway, indicating how it is that messages are passed to the brain. It is, of course, the processing of these messages in the brain which gives us our picture of the world of sound. Please refer to Figure 1.

The Outer Ear

The outer ear consists of a trumpet-shaped, partially cartilaginous flange called the pinna. This is the variable-sized flap at the side of the head attached by ligaments and muscles. It includes a resonant cavity called the concha and a canal or 'external auditory meatus' which leads to the eardrum, or tympanic membrane. The external auditory meatus has sebaceous glands (ceruminous glands) for the secretion of cerumen (wax) which helps to keep the ear clean and clear of foreign bodies. In the context of deafness and the use of hearing aids it is important to realise that the pinna and concha support the earmould which delivers sound to the ear from a hearing aid. Scrutiny of Figure 1. also reveals that

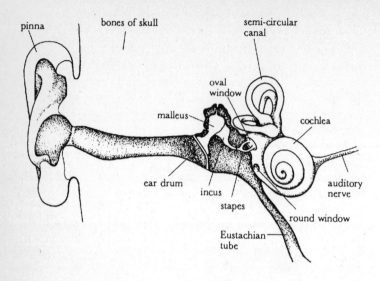

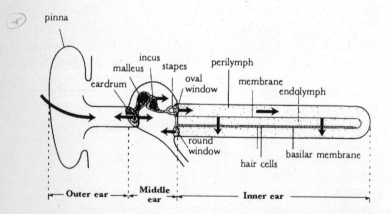

Figure 1. Diagrams of the hearing mechanism. Above: the human ear. Below: diagrammatic section through the ear; with cochlea unwound. Reproduced from *Biology, GCSE Edition* by Geoff and Mary Jones (Cambridge University Press, 1987) by kind permission of Geoff Jones.

the ear canal has both a cartilaginous and a bony section. It is important that an earmould does not fit down the ear canal past the junction of the cartilaginous and bony sections. Hairs in the outer third of the ear canal serve to catch debris and prevent it passing right down the ear canal and building up, ultimately to block the canal and interfere with the passage of sound. Secretions in the ear canal serve to maintain a very steady temperature/humidity balance in the area near to the tympanic membrane.

The outer ear is also important in aiding sound localisation, the most important cues being intensity and timing differences in the sound-waves which strike the two ears. For example, the sound-waves from the right, which strike the right ear first, are more intense at that ear. The convolutions of the pinna also cause sounds to reflect from its surfaces and this helps the listener to decide whether a sound is coming from directly in front, behind or above.

The Middle Ear
The middle ear is a small air-filled cavity beyond the tympanic membrane which contains three tiny bones or ossicles. These bones are known as the malleus, incus and stapes. They are suspended across the middle ear cavity from eardrum to a flexible window, the oval window, situated in the bony wall which separates middle ear and inner ear. The malleus is embedded in the eardrum. The incus is connected to the malleus at one end and to the stapes at the other. The footplate of the stapes fits snugly against the oval window. A second membrane-covered window, called the round window because of its shape, is situated in the wall of the inner ear. One of the functions of the ossicles is to apply greater force to one window, the oval window. As we shall see later, this is important if the inner ear is to be able to do its job properly.

The wall of the middle ear also provides an opening to the *Eustachian tube,* which is a narrow tube running from the nasopharynx to the middle ear. It is normally closed but opens to allow pressure equalisation in the middle ear upon blowing the nose or swallowing.

The job of the middle ear is to pass sound energy, which originates at a source outside the ear, from the external auditory meatus to the inner ear which is filled with relatively dense liquids.

THE CONDUCTIVE PATHWAY (OUTER AND MIDDLE EAR)
If one imagines a sound-wave travelling from source, for example a musical instrument, to a receiver, the ear, it becomes possible to appreciate the marvellous way in which nature has equipped us so that we are able to perceive such sounds and derive pleasure from them. When a source emits sound it basically sets up vibration in the surrounding medium. Sound is a form of energy produced whenever an object is set into vibration. In our world this medium is the gaseous medium of air and it is via the air molecules that sound energy (that which produces vibration) passes from source to receiver. The vibrating source sets up tiny disturbances in the surrounding medium—these disturbances being increases and decreases of air pressure relative to normal ambient pressure. The pressure changes are tiny—for example, the pressure change induced by a 'just audible' tone in the mid-frequency region (1500 Hertz) is 20 units of air pressure (μPa), while we live under an air pressure of 100,000Pa. Very painful sounds have pressure of about 200Pa.

As the sound-wave travels through the medium, the sound energy is being passed on by the air molecules via vibration. Eventually the sound-wave will arrive at a listener. From the viewpoint of a sound-wave it simply impinges upon a funnel (the pinna) which acts to feed the sound-wave down a natural tube (the ear canal) to a terminating membrane, the tympanic membrane, which is able to vibrate in response to the sound pressure variation and hence 'pass on' the sound energy via mechanical vibration.

Because the outer ear is surrounded by the skull and has a trumpet like canal, sound-waves are enhanced on arrival at the eardrum. Technically we would say that this is caused by head baffle and ear canal resonance. These two effects combine to produce a 10 to 15 decibel (dB) enhancement in the frequency region 1.5 to 7 kiloHertz (kHz). The head-baffle effects are centred around 5kHz, the ear canal resonance around 2.6kHz.

If a person is to hear sounds it is necessary for the vibrations in the air to be translated into vibrations in the liquid in the inner ear. This in turn produces electro-chemical activity in the auditory nerve fibres. This can only be achieved effectively by means of the *conductive pathway* of the ear.

One may ask why it is necessary to have a conductive pathway. Why not simply place the cochlea with oval and round windows at the entrance to the ear canal and let the air molecules pass on their acoustic energy directly to the perilymph (one of the two principal liquids of the inner ear) via the oval window? The problem would be that very little energy would pass to the perilymph molecules. It would be much like trying to set a trampoline into vibration by hitting it with a balloon. Most of the energy would be reflected. The problem stems from the fact that air is a compressible gas with relatively light molecules while perilymph is incompressible and much denser. It is necessary to boost the incoming sound-wave (sound pressure) so that an effective transfer of energy to a liquid medium is achieved. In effect, an acoustic transformer is required to match the low-impedance air medium with the high-impedance liquid medium. The conductive pathway is specially suited to achieve this objective.

It does this in two principal ways. Firstly, there is considerable difference between the surface areas of the oval window and of the tympanic membrane to which it is directly linked by the ossicles. The effective area of the tympanic membrane is about eighteen times that of the oval window. Since the same amount of energy is being transferred from a large area to a small one, the pressure per unit area is increased (just as it is increased when a woman changes her flat-heeled shoes to stilettos, as the cork floor readily shows!). The pressure is increased in the same proportion as the ratio of the two areas, so in the case of the middle ear there is an eighteen-times increase in pressure at the oval window simply because the tympanic membrane is that much larger.

Secondly, the effect is further enhanced by the anatomical properties of the ossicles. These may be considered as a series of levers. Since the length of the manubrium and neck of the malleus is longer than the long process of the incus, a mechanical advantage of 1.3 results. This increases the pressure at the stapes by a further factor of 1.3 so that overall boost to sound pressure at the stapes footplate is approximately 23 times (i.e. 18 x 1.3). In decibels this is approximately equivalent to 27dB.

The net result is that the pressure at the stapes footplate is enhanced so that a reasonable degree of impedance matching occurs. The work of Zwislocki suggests that it is because of the transfer function of the conductive system that our ears are most sensitive in the mid-frequency region.

The Inner Ear
The inner ear is a complicated arrangement of tubes filled with watery fluid. Part of this arrangement, the *cochlea,* is concerned with hearing; and part, the *utricle* and *semi-circular canals,* with our sense of balance.

THE COCHLEA
The cochlea lies just beyond the middle ear cavity and is shaped like a snail shell of two-and-a-half turns. The oval window is situated in the outer wall of its bony casing.The cochlea is divided into three chambers: scala vestibuli, scala tympani and cochlear duct. The two scalae are in effect parallel circular stairways within the spiral, the upper scala vestibuli, the lower scala tympani. Both contain a fluid, perilymph, which resembles cerebrospinal fluid. They join at the helicotrema at the top of the spiral. The upper scala connects to the oval window, the lower scala to the round window, the second membrane in the party wall between the middle ear and cochlea.This membrane is slightly smaller and more compliant than the oval window.

The cochlear duct is a wedge-shaped compartment lying between the scalae. It contains the fluid endolymph which resembles intracellular fluid.There is no direct connection between the perilymph and endolymph. The cochlear duct contains the sensory nerve endings of the auditory nerve embedded in two membranes—the *basilar* and *tectorial* membranes. There are thought to be approximately 30,000 nerve endings—the hair cells—lying along the cochlear duct. It is generally agreed that the arrangement of the hair cells on the basilar membrane, and the structure of the latter contribute substantially to pitch discrimination in the cochlear duct. Higher-pitched sounds are resolved by the nerve fibre closer to the oval window and sounds of lower pitch by fibres farther along the membrane towards the helicotrema. All of the fibres come together in a bunch as they leave the cochlea and constitute the nerve of hearing which conveys information to the auditory cortex.

Vibrations that are transmitted to the oval window by the footplate of the stapes in the middle ear set up vibrations in the perilymph which surrounds the membranous labyrinth containing the end organs of hearing and balance in the inner ear. The vibrations spread upward in the scala vestibuli, are transmitted through *Reissner's membrane* to the endolymph and thence through the basilar membrane to the scala tympani where they pass downward to the round window. The vibrations of the round window therefore occur a fraction of a second later and in the opposite direction (opposite phase) to that of the oval window. The vibrations of the basilar membrane cause a pull or shearing force on the hair cells attached to the tectorial membrane. This action transforms the fluid vibratory energy into electrical impulses that stimulate the fibres of the acoustic nerve (eighth cranial nerve) for onward transmission to the brain. The cochlea and the auditory nerve endings in the duct form part of the *sensorineural pathway* of sound to the brain.

Theories about the Hearing Mechanism
Most hearing theories put forward over the years can be placed into one of two general types:
   •*Space pattern theory*. Here it is assumed that the frequency information of the incoming sound-wave is translated into a

spatial pattern on the basilar membrane. Different areas of this membrane are stimulated by different frequencies. The brain thus receives impulses which provide information on *time* features, but it does so by means of the *location* of the nerves which are stimulated.

• *Time pattern theory*. Here it is assumed that the time features are transmitted directly to the brain.

Harvey Fletcher, a former Director of Physical Research at Bell Telephone Laboratories, put forward the suggestion that both of the effects described above aid humans in interpreting the sounds which they hear. He suggested that therefore a *space-time pattern theory* of hearing best expressed the conception. This theory is explained in detail in *Speech and Hearing in Communication* (Van Nostrand, Princeton, New Jersey, 1953). He argues that the pitch of a tone is determined both by the position of its maximum stimulation on the basilar membrane and by the time pattern sent to the brain, the former being probably more important for the high tones and the latter for low tones. Loudness is dependent upon the number of nerve impulses per second reaching the brain and is probably identified by the length of the stimulated area of the basilar membrane. This stimulation is carried to the brain and forms a portion of excited brain matter of a definite size. This size determines our sensation of the loudness of the tone.

So the time-sequence pattern in the air is converted to space pattern on the basilar membrane. The nerve endings are excited in such a way that the space pattern is transferred to the brain and produces two similar patterns, one on the left side and one on the right side. Enough of the time pattern in the air is sent to each of these stimulated areas to make time sequence of maximum stimulation detectable.

WHAT GOES WRONG WITH HEARING IN CHILDREN AND CAN IT BE CURED?

For a child to have normal hearing, the outer, middle and inner ear must function normally. Hearing impairment arises when disease or abnormality occurs in one or more of these parts. If the problem occurs somewhere along the conductive pathway, i.e. in the outer or middle ear, the resulting deafness is known as a *conductive deafness*. If it occurs in the inner ear it is known as *sensori-neural* or *nerve deafness*. If it occurs in two or more parts of the ear it is called *mixed deafness*.

Conductive Deafness

This type of deafness relates to a 'blockage' or other form of inhibitor of vibration occurring in the outer or middle ear. It generally results in a partial rather than a severe degree of hearing loss. However research has shown that such losses are educationally important and can affect children's language acquisition and school progress if they are present for long periods of time (see Garner[1] for a review of the literature). Children are more likely to suffer from conductive hearing loss in early childhood and, as a result of changes in the shape of the skull due to growth, it becomes less common as they near the age of nine or ten.

Conductive problems are frequently caused by fluid or foreign-body blockages of the outer or middle ear. The blockage results in a dampening of the sound vibration, which in turn makes the sound too quiet to hear. Problems of this sort are frequently amenable to either medical or surgical intervention.

Congenital conductive deafness arises in the womb at the time when the ear is developing. A variety of anomalies can occur including: the complete absence of the outer ear; the auricle being present as a remnant only; occlusion of the ear canal (i.e. the ear canal being closed over with no open tube to the tympanic membrane); and complete absence of ossicles. Children frequently are affected in one ear only, the other being normal. In such cases the usual procedure is for the audiologist to monitor the good ear to ensure that it stays normal. Most children with one good ear do quite well at school providing they are treated sympathetically and given a preferential seat close to the teacher. Of course it is for the surgeon to decide if and when a blocked ear canal should be opened or a reconstruction of the middle ear attempted.

PROBLEMS OF THE OUTER EAR

Wax is by far the commonest cause of obstruction of the external auditory canal and any deafness is usually perceived suddenly when blockage becomes total. Ear wax is a normal secretion from the ceruminous glands and it usually finds its own way out of the ear canal without causing any problems. However the wax is hygroscopic (absorbs water) and a build-up of wax can absorb moisture, swell up and block the ear. Deafness is often noticed after swimming or bathing for this reason. The usual approaches to removal are to soften it with drops (e.g., olive oil) and then to allow it to come out itself or to syringe or suck it out. Parents, or anyone else for that matter, should *not* poke objects such as cotton-wool buds down a child's ear canal. Wax occurs naturally and carries dirt out of the ear canal. It can be a problem with hearing impaired children wearing earmoulds, the earmoulds acting to prevent the free passage of the wax out of the ear. The ears of hearing aid users should be examined frequently for impacted wax.

Foreign bodies are a more common problem than some people may realise. Children have a tendency to put objects in the strangest places! Pieces of matchstick, plastic and ballbearings have been seen by the writer down children's ears. Of course it is unlikely that a foreign body placed in the ear canal, unless it totally blocks the canal, would cause significant hearing loss but there are obvious dangers for the tympanic membrane and the objects allow the build-up of wax around them. This wax dries out (colour goes very dark-brown) and a solid plug of it will cause hearing loss. Any suspicion that a young child has been pushing objects down its ear should encourage the parent to take the child to see a doctor.

PROBLEMS OF THE MIDDLE EAR

The middle ear cavity is filled with air by the opening and closing of the Eustachian tube (as in yawning or swallowing) and it contains the middle ear ossicles which vibrate in response to eardrum vibration. It is vital that the eardrum remains flexible and that the ossicles vibrate freely if sound is to be transmitted efficiently through the middle ear. We will say a little about the eustachian tube shortly but at this point it is important to highlight that if the tube does not work efficiently then conductive deafness can result.

The whole of the middle ear cleft is lined by a continuous layer of mucous membrane, and acute infections *(acute otitis media)* can spread very rapidly over the whole surface of the cleft. By far the commonest cause of acute inflammations in the cleft is the common cold but any upper respiratory tract infection can spread to this area. Acute infections of the cleft occur most frequently in young children and are often associated with infections of the adenoids and tonsils.

The role of the eustachian tube is a key one since infection here, or blockage (perhaps by infected adenoids), will prevent the entry of air to the middle ear. When blockage of the tube persists the air pressure in the middle ear drops and a watery fluid flows from the mucosal lining of the cleft into the middle ear. The negative middle ear pressure causes a stiffening of the tympanic membrane, and the fluid, which may become infected and thick, severely dampens the movement of the ossicles.

The problems faced by the ossicles can be likened to that of a person standing in a swimming pool. That person would find it relatively easy to walk in an empty pool, but if that pool were filled with water it would be far more difficult to move. So it is for the middle ear ossicles, and therefore *middle ear effusion* results in a conductive hearing impairment.

The treatment of middle-ear deafness resulting from effusion varies according to its severity and the cause of the underlying problem. It has been found that a large majority of cases clear spontaneously without treatment, or with simple treatment such as a course of medicine from the child`s GP (e.g., decongestant, nasal spray). Other children may require the help of the ENT surgeon who may decide to perform an operation. This operation will likely have two aims in view: firstly, to restore normal eustachian tube function and secondly, to remove any middle ear fluid (or 'glue' the name for the fluid when it has become very thick). The fluid is drained by making a tiny slit in the tympanic membrane and then sucking out the fluid *(paracentesis)*. If the surgeon believes that normal tubal function may not have been restored a small teflon tube *(grommet)* may be surgically inserted into the tympanic membrane in order to allow air to pass through it into the middle ear (see Plate 1). The grommets can be of different types and may stay in the ear for a period up to two years. Some types simply fall out and flow out of the ear with wax; others must be removed, when appropriate, by the surgeon. On occasion it is decided that it is enlargement of the adenoids which is causing the blockage of the tube and these will be removed at the same time.

Some children who undergo surgery require a repeat operation but in many cases the problem is resolved by one operation and does not occur again.

Down's syndrome is worth mentioning in the context of conductive hearing loss since many studies have shown that children with this condition are particularly vulnerable to middle-ear dysfunction. They have very narrow ear canals and are prone to allergic reactions to the mucosal lining of the upper respiratory tract and middle-ear cleft. Such children should always be examined by an audiologist.

Spotting the Signs of Conductive Deafness in the Classroom

We are often asked by mainstream teachers how they might spot the child with a conductive hearing loss. Apart from the findings of hearing and impedance tests the following may be seen in the classroom:

1   One of the most obvious signs is the child who appears 'catarrhal' or is a mouth breather and has frequent short absences with coughs, colds or sore throats. The child may also complain of earache or 'popping' or 'full' sensations in the ear. Check the attendance register and if this fits with other observations the matter should be reported to the service for hearing-impaired children.

2 The child frequently mishears in the classroom or perhaps appears to be a daydreamer or is more subject to distraction than other children.

3 The child may have difficulty in following instructions, gets the wrong idea, or watches and follows other children. This situation would normally be worse in adverse noise conditions. It may also make the child less interested in activities which require concentration e.g., listening to a story. A further manifestation might be aggressive or bad-tempered behaviour.

4 If the child 'hears' but doesn't 'hear' then it is likely that the he is responding to the louder low frequency sounds but is not following and understanding the 'messages' which are heavily dependent on the quieter high frequency parts of speech such as 's', 'p', and 't'.

5 A more difficult one to tie to deafness is the fact that the child may be more demanding of your attention and press for more individual help since in these situations you will be closer to him and therefore what you say will be heard better than when you are addressing the whole class. This child would also wish to be closer to any television or tape recorder.

6 You occasionally may notice that a child is speaking much more quietly than usual.

If teachers are in any way suspicious that a child does not hear properly then they should not hesitate in seeking specialist advice. A hearing loss is too serious a problem to be ignored.

It is quite natural for teachers of ordinary children to be worried about having a hearing impaired child in their class, particularly if they are given no additional help. We would also have to say that the help provided by services for hearing impaired children is very variable in both amount and quality. In Chapter 3 we outline the main areas of knowledge needed by mainstream teachers.

SENSORI-NEURAL DEAFNESS

Sensori-neural hearing impairments are usually divided into two types: those occurring prior to birth i.e. as a result of hereditary factors or infections whilst the baby is in the womb, and those where the child has a perfectly normal hearing mechanism at birth but is later attacked by some damaging infection or trauma e.g., meningitis. These are termed *congenital* and *acquired* respectively.

Congenital Sensori-Neural Deafness

Congenital sensori-neural deafness is usually divided into three further sub-groups : the hereditary group, due to genetic factors; the prenatal group, resulting from damage to the inner ear of the baby as it develops in the womb; and the peri-natal, due to one or more factors which may affect the baby at or around the time of birth.

Hereditary Deafness

Hereditary deafness is the term used when the baby inherits the deafness from the parents. When a baby is conceived it receives certain 'characters' from its parents which are carried inside each cell on the *chromosomes*. Human cells carry 23 chromosomes—children receive 23 from each parent which then pair up. The 'characters' carried by the chromosomes determine all our physical functions, including hearing. One of each pair of characters is *dominant* and governs the hearing (or other function) of the child and the weaker character (called the *recessive)* has no influence.

If we consider only the question of hearing, normally hearing people generally carry two similar characters, both of which are consistent with normal hearing. It is possible, however, for a parent to be a carrier of a recessive hearing character which produces sensori-neural deafness even though he or she has normal hearing. This occurs when the parents, neither deaf themselves but each carrying a recessive character for deafness, produce children. They have approximately a 25 per cent chance of producing a deaf child. As these deafnesses are unpredictable it is difficult to be certain but some authors have argued that recessive genetic deafness accounts for 50 per cent or more of all sensori-neural deafness.

It is sometimes possible from detailed investigations of a family to trace family-linked deafness through generation to generation. In such cases the parents passing on the hearing defect are hearing impaired themselves and the chances of conceiving a hearing impaired child are greater (approximately 50 per cent risk). The hearing impaired person in such cases carries a dominant deafness gene.

One pair of the 23 pairs of chromosomes determines the sex of the child. The other 22 are known as *autosomes* and it is generally the case that information concerned with hearing function will be carried by the autosomes. It has, however, been found that sex-linked deafness does occasionally occur.

It is important to appreciate that children can inherit single or multiple abnormalities or characteristics including deafness. Some of these may group themselves together and such groups are generally known as *syndromes:* collections of characteristics that are passed on together through families. One such syndrome is Waardenburg`s syndrome. The characteristic features of this syndrome are white 'forelock' and heterochromia iridium (one eye brown and the other blue).

Sometimes parents are advised that the cause of their child's deafness is 'unknown'. This rather broad term is somewhat deceptive, since it is in fact more precise than it first appears. This is because it should be known that the deafness does *not* have certain causes; so an 'unknown' deafness may for example be known *not to have been caused* by maternal rubella or anoxia or cytomegalovirus. By eliminating the possibilities in this way one can come to the conclusion that a likely cause may be hereditary factors. Statistical analyses strongly suggest that the great majority of occurrences of deafness of unknown cause are indeed inherited. For this reason where parents are told that the cause of their child's hearing impairment is unknown, the advice of a genetic counsellor should sought. This doctor will probably be based in a hospital and be a specialist in the study of heredity. She or he will be able to offer guidance on the likelihood of the deafness being inherited, and on the chances that further children will inherit the deafness too. Such counselling will be particularly important if and when the child itself considers starting a family. However, the seeking of such advice should be done as early as possible since if it is left until the child grows up it may not be possible for the geneticist to track down sufficient information to be really helpful.

PRE-NATAL SENSORI-NEURAL DEAFNESS
It is possible for the mother to contract German measles (rubella virus) for the first time during her pregnancy. If this happens, the virus is passed on and infects the baby. As far as the mother is concerned, she suffers no more than minor discomfort from a slight fever and a rash. However, the consequences for the unborn baby can be catastrophic. The virus can cause multiple handicaps in babies including sensori-neural deafness, blindness, mental retardation and heart defects.

The risk of rubella infection damaging an unborn baby depends very much upon the time during the pregnancy when the infection occurs. The risk is known to be greatest during the first 12 to 16 weeks of pregnancy and to decline thereafter. The sensori-neural deafness results from the fact that the virus destroys part of the cochlea especially during periods of rapid development.

The saddest feature is that rubella is an almost entirely preventable infection (inoculation is about 95 per cent effective). The inoculation is freely available and is offered to all girls between the ages of 11 and 14 through the School Health Service. It is also available to anyone else, particularly women in child-bearing years, from general practitioners. However, it should *not* be given *during* pregnancy, or within three months of intended conception. It is also considered desirable that it should be delayed if a blood transfusion has been performed.

The policy in the United Kingdom is now to try to protect the whole female population from this virus *before* they have children. Official figures indicate that the immunisation take-up rate is improving. In 1978 it was 55 per cent. By 1983 this had risen to 84 per cent, but with a regional variation of 75 to 92 per cent. The most recent estimates suggest a take-up rate of 90 per cent. However there is no room for complacency.

Readers may be interested in the findings of two studies into the causes of sensori-neural deafness in children. Both were carried out in Greater Manchester, the first by Taylor, covering all children born between 1975–8, and the second by Newton, covering 1977–80. In the first, 33 per cent of children with bilateral sensori-neural deafness of greater than 80dBHL were deafened by rubella. The figure for the second study was 8.6 per cent. It might be thought that an increase in the take-up of rubella immunisation was entirely responsible for the reduction in incidence of rubella handicapped children, but therapeutic abortions also increased very significantly during the same period, so mothers who had contracted rubella were clearly being advised, or were much more willing, to terminate the pregnancy. It is quite clear to us that the way to reduce the number of rubella-handicapped children is for *all* to take up the vaccine. Lastly, some women 'lose' their protection (antibodies) against rubella. Blood tests can indicate whether this is in fact the case and it is our view that these should be carried out *prior to starting a family*.

Some other viral infections present during pregnancy, such as cytomegalovirus, have been shown to give rise to deafness in some children.

PERI-NATAL SENSORI-NEURAL DEAFNESS

Low birth-weight. Sensori-neural deafness does occur in a small number of low-birth-weight babies e.g., in cases of severe *prematurity*. However, with better facilities and improved infant care this is becoming increasingly rare.

Anoxia. During a long and difficult labour, or soon after a difficult birth, it is possible for a baby to become short of oxygen. This sometimes has been believed to cause hearing impairment, although the exact mechanisms are not identified. In studies at Manchester University it was found that children whose heart actually stopped beating at birth, were more at risk with regard to hearing than children with classical anoxia. What is greatly encouraging is that anoxia is becoming increasingly rare, because of great strides in the care of 'at risk' babies around the time of birth.

Neonatal jaundice.   At birth jaundice may occur owing to the relative immaturity of the baby's liver, coupled with the breakdown of red blood cells as the cell count falls from seven to five million per cubic millimetre in the first few weeks of life. This problem will obviously be more significant in the less developed premature baby. A substance known as bilirubin is produced as a result of the breakdown of the red blood cells and bilirubin passes from the blood to the liver to be excreted. Any blockage or failure of the excretory system results in an accumulation of bilirubin in the blood. When this happens the baby turns yellow and is said to be jaundiced. Deafness as a result of high levels of bilirubin occurs because of damage to the nerve of hearing at the brain stem. The condition is called *kernicterus*. Treatment is by phototherapy and in severe cases by blood transfusion.

Rhesus incompatibility.   Where an individual's blood contains a substance called the Rhesus factor (D) it is known as 'Rhesus positive blood'. If it does not contain this factor it is known as 'Rhesus negative'. Some people are born with Rhesus positive blood (85 per cent), the remainder have Rhesus negative blood. The Rhesus factor is carried in the red blood cells. If a Rhesus negative woman is sensitised (i.e. given Rhesus positive blood), she will produce an anti-Rhesus (or anti-D) factor.

This can give rise to a problem when a Rhesus negative mother is carrying a Rhesus positive baby. During the time the baby is in the womb, the placenta allows the passage of nutrients to the baby and the removal of waste products. It does not, however, in normal circumstances, allow the passage of red cells from one circulation to the other. However, if the maternal circulation contains anti-D, this can pass through the placenta into the baby's circulation where it will meet D cells. These will be destroyed releasing bilirubin into the child's blood stream. If there is a high concentration of anti-D present, then the life of the baby will be threatened. If the baby is born alive it will be severely jaundiced and will require exchange transfusions and phototherapy.

Anti-D may develop in a Rhesus negative woman following a pregnancy in which the child is Rhesus positive, without any obvious Rhesus positive transfusion having been given at any time. It is thought that slight placental damage resulting in some of the baby's Rhesus positive cells entering the maternal circulation accounts for this situation. This would not affect the child in question, but would have serious implications for any subsequent Rhesus positive pregnancies.

Nowadays the situation can be remedied by injecting anti-D to Rhesus negative women immediately after child-birth, to destroy any possible Rhesus positive cells from the baby which may have entered the maternal circulation during the separation of the baby's placenta and the mother's uterus. If this is not done then the mother will be sensitised and develop her own anti-D which will persist and threaten any subsequent pregnancy. The injected anti-D will have disappeared by then.

Before the development of the anti-D injection the Rhesus factor accounted for a significant number of sensori-neural deaf children. Now such cases are rare.

ACQUIRED SENSORI-NEURAL DEAFNESS IN CHILDREN

Viruses

Several viral infections are reported as causing sensori-neural deafness. Although it is rare, measles has been reported as such a virus. Mumps occasionally causes hearing defect, but this almost always affects only one ear, the other being left perfectly normal. This unilateral deafness may go undetected for a long time. Influenza has also been linked with deafness.

In all the above cases the damage appears to arise in the cochlea and the loss is sudden at the time of infection.

Meningitis

This is an inflammation of the membrane covering the brain due to bacterial or viral infection. It is probably the most common cause of significant acquired sensori-neural deafness in children. The hearing loss is often very severe indeed.

Damage to the hearing mechanism usually occurs in the cochlea, although higher centres along the acoustic nerve may also be affected. The incidence of hearing loss as a result of meningitis has been drastically reduced by antibiotic therapy. In the case of bacterial meningitis, it is now estimated that as few as 3 to 5 per cent of children affected are likely to have hearing problems.

At one time tubercular meningitis, which is now very rare in Britain, was treated with an antibiotic called streptomycin. This drug itself is now known to be a cause of sensori-neural deafness when taken in large quantities. Alternative drugs are therefore used in such cases, and only a drastically reduced dosage of streptomycin, if any at all.

AIDS TO HEARING WITH DIFFERENT FORMS OF DEAFNESS

Hearing Aids

We have already indicated that when the hearing loss is conductive in origin the preferred approach is likely to be medical (use of medicines) or surgical (surgical attempts to ensure an aerated middle ear or to ensure the free passage of sounds through the outer and middle ear structures). It is the view of the present authors that where the conductive hearing loss is marked and long-standing then hearing aids should be fitted and the hearing loss monitored very frequently. Evidence of large studies on conductive hearing loss have generally been equivocal about the long-term effects but we both have seen in clinic many children suffering quite severe social and educational effects of such losses. For the audiologist the fitting is relatively simple and the benefits are immediate. For Downs syndrome children where conductive problems are very common and very difficult to remedy long term fittings have been made very successfully.

Until recently the only amplification available for sensori-neural deafness was via hearing aids and these are still the preferred choice of system for the vast majority of children. The great majority of children have remaining hearing which is amenable to stimulation with hearing aids. This hearing is often present over a relatively wide spread of frequencies and for this the hearing aid is to be preferred to other forms of stimulation.

Cochlear Implants

There is increasing use of cochlear implants with a population of *totally deaf* children and this practice is likely to grow in the United Kingdom. The cochlear implant is an electronic device which directly stimulates the child's auditory nerve (see Plate II). It is usually the hair cells in the cochlear duct which convert vibrations into electrical stimuli which are then picked up by the auditory nerve and transmitted to the brain. The purpose of the cochlear implant is to transmit sound information so that it stimulates the auditory nerve directly. In all cochlear implant systems sounds are collected by an external microphone and are then converted to electrical signals which are passed to a 'speech processor'. The processor passes on the signals to the electrode array within the implant.

Single– and multi-channel systems have been produced for implantation. As the name suggests, the multi-channel system has more than one electrode, each electrode delivering different information to the auditory nerve. The implant may be fitted in a variety of places including outside the cochlea on the promontory or near the oval window. Implants placed beyond the oval window are likely to be placed in the scala tympani or possibly directly at the auditory nerve.

Probably the most widely used multi-channel device is that developed at the University of Melbourne by Professor Graham Clark and his team. In this device low frequency signals are directed towards the apex of the cochlear duct, which is more sensitive to lower frequencies, and higher frequencies are directed towards the basal area.

Prior to fitting an implant the patients undergo a very detailed audiological and medical examination including X-rays of the temporal bone and tests to indicate whether the auditory nerve is still intact.

Post-operatively an intensive testing and rehabilitation programme is carried out. The levels of electrical stimulation are set and the channels of the speech processor are programmed. Parents and others involved with pre-lingually deaf children should be aware that fitting an implant does not immediately 'turn on' normal speech and language, any more than does a conventional hearing aid. The child must undergo a long period of habilitation and learn to make use of the sounds it hears through the processor. This can take many years. The key thing to remember is that the implant is much like a hearing aid except that the signals from the hearing aid are passed through the conventional channels of the outer, middle ear, cochlea and on to the auditory nerve, whereas the implant passes the signals directly to the nerve of hearing. The hearing aid tries to use the remains of a damaged but fantastically sophisticated sound analyser, the implant tries to bypass that with an as yet relatively unsophisticated device. Most professionals would agree that the implant only becomes the device of choice when it has been clearly demonstrated that the patient has no usable hearing.

References

1 Garner M., 'The Conductively Deaf Child – Our Problem', *J. Brit Assn. Teachers of the Deaf*, (9) 4, (1985) pp. 95–100

Useful Reading

Ballantyne, J.C., *Deafness*, Churchill, London. This text offers further detail on the causes and treatment of conductive deafness.

Denes, P.B. and Pinson, E.N., *The Speech Chain*, Bell Telephone Laboratories, 1963. Selected areas. This text is now old but still good in several areas.

Nolan, M. and Tucker, I.G., *'The Hearing Impaired Child and the Family'*, 2nd edn., Souvenir Press, London, 1988. See pp. 20ff for a more detailed but simple description of the genetic features of recessive deafness.

Pickles, J.O., *An Introduction to the Physiology of Hearing*, Academic Press, 1982. Selected areas.

Rosenberg, M., 'Sound and Hearing', *Studies in Biology*, no. 145, Edward Arnold Publishers, 1982.

Tucker, I.G. and Nolan, M., *Educational Audiology*, Chapter 1, Croom Helm, 1984.

2 Understanding Amplification

Hearing aids are instruments which amplify sound. They do not restore hearing. If a person has a hearing loss that results in sounds being distorted, and this applies to almost everybody who has a sensori-neural loss, hearing aids will not be able to correct this; they simply make the distorted sound louder. In spite of this they are nevertheless the lifeline which enables a hearing impaired person to remain in contact with people around them. We cannot stress sufficiently the importance of hearing impaired children being provided with properly fitted, well maintained, high quality hearing aids and being trained in their use. Consistent use of optimum amplification by a child from the earliest possible time and exposure to normal language patterns almost always results in that child developing an understanding of spoken language and an ability to talk intelligibly by the time he or she enters adulthood.

The raw material that a hearing aid processes is sound. Sound is a form of energy that arises as the result of vibrations occurring. These vibrations may occur in solids, liquids or gases. In the normal process of hearing in humans, these vibrations are carried through the air to the ear, which responds by sending signals to the brain, which then 'hears' them as sound. The human ear does not respond to all forms of vibration. So there are some types of 'sound', i.e. the energy produced by vibration, which we cannot hear—ultrasound for example. There are several aspects of sound which are important to hearing aid users, but the two most important relate to the pitch and loudness of sounds. Pitch and loudness are our subjective interpretations of the properties of a particular sound. Since they are subjective they cannot be measured directly. However, the aspects of sound which give rise to these subjective sensations can be.

Frequency is the measure of the rate of vibration and is simply a measure of the number of times something vibrates

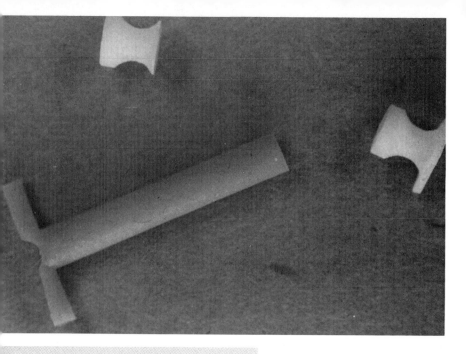

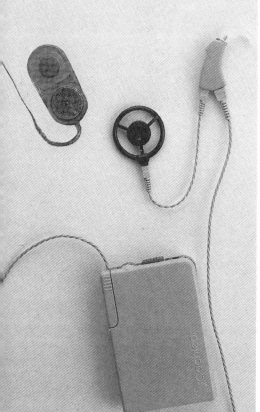

I Two grommets and a 'T' Tube.

II Nucleus cochlear Implant
Courtesy of Cochlear AG,
London.

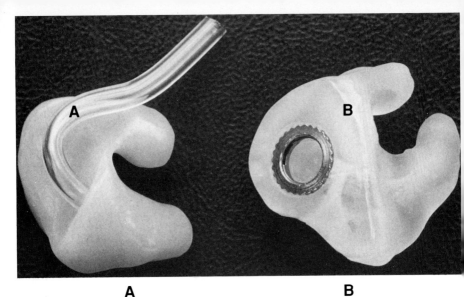

A   **B**

III Two types of earmould.
Left: Mould for ear-level aid.   *Right:* Mould for body-worn aid.

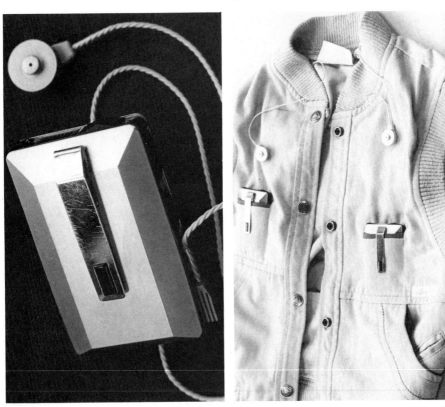

IV *Left:* A) A body-worn hearing aid. *Right:* B) Waistcoat adapted for use as a harness

each second. The unit of measurement is Hertz (Hz) and its multiples. A kiloHertz (kHz) is a thousand vibrations per second and a megaHertz (MHz) a million. The faster something vibrates, i.e. the higher the frequency, the higher pitched a sound becomes. So high frequency gives rise to high pitch, low frequency to low pitched sounds. As a point of reference, middle 'C' on a piano has a frequency of 256Hz. For a note an octave above, the frequency is doubled, so 'C' above middle 'C' has a frequency of 512Hz, and so on.

Loudness is dependent upon sound pressure level (SPL), which is measured in decibels—dB(SPL). When something which is surrounded by air vibrates, it causes pressure variations in the air around it. These pressure variations are passed on as the air molecules themselves are set into vibration. It is these variations in air pressure which travel to the ear and which the ear and the brain interpret as sound. The more vigorous a vibration, the greater the variations in air pressure, the greater the energy transmitted and the greater the decibel count. Sounds with a high decibel level are perceived as being louder than those with a low decibel level. In human terms quiet sounds have a decibel level of 20-30dB(SPL), whereas loud sounds have levels of 80dB(SPL) or more. Normal conversation takes place at a level of about 60db(SPL). One important feature of the sound pressure level scale is that it is a scale of ratios—a logarithmic scale. A 20dB increase in sound pressure level means a tenfold increase in air pressure variation. So 40dB(SPL) is not twice the air pressure change of 20dB(SPL), it is ten times. This also means in air pressure terms that the 20dB difference between 80dB(SPL) and 100db(SPL) is very much greater than the difference between 20dB(SPL) and 40dB(SPL). For those who require it, this subject is covered in greater depth in *Educational Audiology.*[1]

WHAT DO HEARING AIDS DO?

Hearing aids are designed to make the sound pressure level at the eardrum of the wearer greater than it would be without the aid. In other words they make sounds louder. They do this by picking up sound with a microphone, amplifying it, and sending the amplified sound to a receiver or headphone which is attached in some way to the ear. Hearing aids cannot correct any damage which an ear may have suffered, but they may be able to overcome or minimise some of the effects of that damage. Hearing aids are not high fidelity instruments. They are not able to reproduce with great accuracy the sounds in the environment which they amplify. This is largely due to the constraints imposed by size. If hearing aids are to be worn comfortably for long periods of time they cannot be too big or cumbersome. The smaller the aid, the more difficult it is to reproduce sounds accurately at the high levels of amplification required. Even with quite large instruments, such as those which use headphones, it is not possible to achieve high fidelity at the high sound levels needed. So in the sense that hearing aids do not reproduce all sounds accurately we can say that they impose their own form of distortion on the sound being delivered to the ear.

It is important, therefore, that we should be able to measure how well hearing aids perform. By how much do they amplify sound, and how accurately do they do it? It is here that the individual differences between aids emerge; some do some things better than others. We need to know this when we select aids for young children especially, since often they are not able to tell us how good they find a particular aid. While we deal with the electro-acoustic measurement of hearing aid performance later in this chapter, it is important first to understand some of the jargon which is used to describe hearing aids.

Gain is the term used to describe the amount by which an aid amplifies a particular sound. If we measure the sound pressure level of the input sound at the microphone of an aid, and then compare it with the sound pressure level emerging from its receiver, we can determine by how much it has been increased. This increase is called the gain. So if the input is 60dB(SPL) and the output is 100dB(SPL), there has been a gain of 40dB. Because a hearing aid is not completely accurate in the way it reproduces sound, it will give more gain to some frequencies than others. Therefore, when we describe the gain of a hearing aid we must indicate which frequency we are referring to. So we talk about the gain at 1000Hz being 45dB. Sometimes it is more convenient to take the gain of an aid at a number of frequencies and calculate an average. This probably gives a more realistic indication of the aid's capabilities. There are one or two agreed ways of doing this, differing only in the frequencies chosen to form the basis for the average: Gain(HAIC) and Gain(ANSI) are two examples. For the purposes of such specifications the volume control of the aid is always turned up to maximum. This is sometimes called 'full-on' gain. A moderately-powered hearing aid will have a gain of between 20dB to 30dB, whereas some high-power aids have a gain approaching 90dB.

Maximum output is the term used to describe the maximum sound pressure level that an aid is capable of delivering. The output is what comes out of an aid's receiver. Just as you cannot turn up the volume of your transistor radio beyond a certain level, a hearing aid clearly cannot carry on delivering a greater and greater volume ad infinitum. Some component or combination of components imposes a limit. This limitation determines the maximum output. Again, the maximum output is likely to vary with frequency, so the frequency or frequencies which have been used to measure the maximum output should be specified. Maximum output should not be confused with gain. Supposing an aid has a maximum output at 250Hz of 110dB(SPL) and a 'full-on' gain at the same frequency of 50dB. If we now put a signal at 250Hz of 50dB(SPL) into the microphone, we would expect to measure an output of 100dB(SPL). By comparing the input with the output we can see that there has been a gain of 50dB. If we now increase level of the input signal to 110dB(SPL), the output level will be limited to 110dB(SPL) because that is all the aid can deliver at that frequency. By comparing the input with the output we can see that there has been no increase, so the gain is 0dB, even though the volume control of the aid has remained at maximum! This interaction between gain and maximum output is a very important consideration when selecting hearing aids for children. It is usual to show the maximum output of a hearing aid in graph form, by drawing a curve through the points of maximum output at each frequency (see Figure 2). Hearing aids of moderate power will have a maximum output of perhaps 115dB(SPL), with the most powerful exceeding 150dB(SPL).

Input: 90 dB re 20µPa

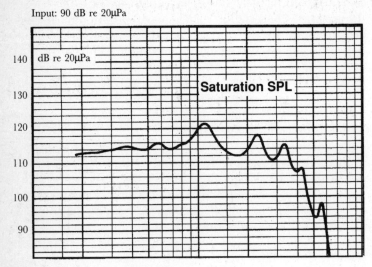

Figure 2. Example of an output curve

Sometimes it is desirable to limit the output of a hearing aid to a level below that of its maximum output. This can be done electronically on some aids which are fitted with internal controls for this purpose. This is usually referred to as output limitation.

The *frequency response* is the other main measure of a hearing aid's performance. As we said above, hearing aids do not give the same amount of gain to each frequency; some are amplified more than others. It is important to know when choosing an aid for a hearing impaired child which frequencies are given more amplification and which less. If we draw a graph of the relative gain of an aid at each frequency, we produce a *frequency response curve*. Since the purpose of a frequency response curve is to show the *relative* amount of amplification given to each frequency, it is usual for the necessary measurements to be made at a setting other than 'full-on' gain. This is often referred to as the 'reference test gain control position'. The precise setting of the volume control depends on the measurement standard being followed. For example, one such standard requires the volume control of the hearing aid to be adjusted until the gain at 1000Hz is 40dB. Measurements are then made across the full frequency range with the volume control in this position, with an input of 60dB(SPL) at each frequency (see Figure 3).

Input: 60 dB re 20μPa
Gain control: adjusted to 40 dB acoustic gain at 1000 Hz

dB re 20μPa

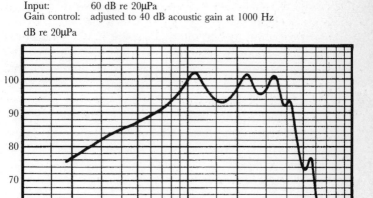

Figure 3. Example of a frequency response curve

Controls

Hearing aids have a range of controls to enable the sound emerging from the receiver to be adjusted to suit the needs of the wearer. These controls may be internal pre-set controls, which are usually set by an audiologist and not intended to be changed once they have been set, and user controls which the user can change at will as the listening conditions around him change. Basically, no matter what manufacturers choose to call them, the controls are of three basic types: those that control the gain, those that control the frequency response, and those that control the maximum output.

GAIN CONTROLS

These controls adjust the volume of the sound for the listener. There is an external control for the wearer to alter. Usually this takes the form of a small numbered wheel. But there may also be an internal pre-set control which effectively limits the range through which the external control operates.

TONE CONTROLS

Tone controls change the frequency response of the aid. These can be both internal and external, though the trend is for them to become mostly internal. There is no standardised form for these controls, although external controls are often labelled 'H', 'N' or 'L' for high frequency emphasis, normal, and low frequency emphasis. Unless indicated otherwise by an educational audiologist, hearing-impaired children should be given the benefit of the widest possible frequency response, and it is particularly important that the low frequencies should not be cut as they frequently are for adults who develop deafness later on in life.

OUTPUT CONTROLS

These controls limit the output of the aid to a pre-determined level. In some hearing aids this may be combined with the volume control, but mostly they are internal pre-set controls. While there are sophisticated variations, output limitation can be one of two broad types, *peak clipping* or *automatic gain control*. Both have their advantages and disadvantages and it is for the audiologist to decide which is the one to use where output limitation is thought to be necessary in the case of a particular individual. Most hearing-impaired children with severe or profound losses do not need output limitation, but for those who do it is essential that it be provided, or rejection of an aid may result.

DIFFERENT TYPES OF AMPLIFICATION SYSTEMS USED BY CHILDREN

Amplification systems used by hearing impaired children are of three main types: those that are worn entirely by the child; those which are used in fixed locations (wearing headphones); and those where part of the system is worn by the child and part by someone else (using transmitters). By far the most common are those worn by the children,—their *personal aids.* Most children will need to wear two, one in each ear. There are three types of these aids: bodyworn, earlevel, and in-the-ear.

Earmoulds

All three types have one thing in common in that they are used in conjunction with an *earmould* which is fitted into the outer ear. The purpose of the earmould is to hold a hearing aid, or receiver of a hearing aid in place and to conduct the amplified sound into the ear canal. Earmoulds are attached to their hearing aids in different ways, either by a short length of acoustic tubing, or by a special clip which fits onto a button receiver used with bodyworn aids (see Plate III). They are made of a variety of materials, they may be clear or opaque, of various colours and of differing degrees of softness. The two important aspects are that they should fit well, and that they should be kept clean. If they are not kept clean, quite apart from hygienic considerations, they may interfere with the quality of the sound reaching the eardrum. If they do not fit well they will cause a high-pitched annoying whistle or howling which is called 'acoustic feedback'. The daily cleaning of earmoulds is easy, but the correction of a poor fit is not. The only answer in this case is for a new mould to be made. Young children quickly outgrow their earmoulds and at some periods of their lives they may need new earmoulds every month or so. This process should be put in train by informing the teacher of the deaf, or audiologist who is overseeing the child's amplification needs, as soon as the whistling starts to occur. With some children the shape of their ears is such that it is difficult to get a well-fitting mould. Where there are such difficulties great care should be taken to get a faithful replica of the ear at the impression stage. If a good mould is still not forthcoming, different mould materials and suppliers should be tried, giving instructions that moulds should be made that are an *exact* and unmodified replica of the impression. Turning down the volume control of a hearing aid will reduce its tendency to whistle, but this strategy should only be adopted as a temporary measure because by doing this you are depriving the child of the amplification he needs.

Personal Aids

BODYWORN AIDS

These aids are the most powerful personal aids available. They are excellent aids to use with young profoundly hearing impaired children. Sometimes called pocket aids, they consist of a small box which houses the electronics (a microphone, the amplifier and its controls), and a button-like receiver which is held into the ear by a custom-made earmould and connected to the amplifier by a lead (see Plate IVa). Because they are bigger, bodyworn aids usually have a better frequency response and more distortion-free power in the low frequencies than the other types available. Also, because the separation between the microphone and the receiver of the aid is relatively large, there is a smaller chance of whistling (acoustic feedback) occurring when high levels of gain are used. With young children they may be a bit of a nuisance to manage unless steps are taken to provide a special harness, or specially adapted clothing, to hold them properly in place, and to keep the leads under control (see Plate IVb). Leads often develop faults with wear and need to be replaced, so teachers and parents need to have spares available. However, the most important consideration is that the child should use the type of amplification he or she will benefit from most, regardless of whether or not the leads are a nuisance! Wearing hearing aids of whatever type should not limit a child's activity in school.

The only place they should not be worn is in the swimming pool.

EAR LEVEL AIDS

Usually known as *post-aural aids,* these hearing aids are worn behind the ear (see Plate Va). They are held in place by the earmould which fits into the ear. All the electronics, the microphone, amplifier and its controls and the receiver are built into the same container. The amplified sound it produces is fed into a sound tube, also called the tone hook, which connects to the tubing of the earmould. Post-aural aids are perhaps more acceptable cosmetically than bodyworn aids and they are probably less prone to damage. The quality of post-aural aids has improved to such an extent over the past decade, that the amplification needs of most children can be met by one or other of the many models available. However, even the very best of these aids do not have the same amount of distortion-free amplification available, in terms of gain or maximum output, as the best bodyworn aids, so they are not suitable for use with every child. There are now very small miniature post-aural aids available for small children (see Plate Vb). These are more easily hidden, and are better at staying put on small soft ears. Clearly their smallness results in some compromises being made in respect of the amplification they provide. Cosmetic considerations are important, but not as important as providing the right kind of amplification. However, for some children, particularly those with less severe losses, they are a welcome and useful addition to the range of aids available.

IN-THE-EAR (ITE) AIDS

These hearing aids fit completely into the outer ear itself. Some may just fit into the ear canal and some will occupy the whole of the 'bowl' or concha of the outer ear. All the electronics and the earmould itself are combined into one piece (see Plate VI). ITE aids are being marketed with great vigour by hearing-aid manufacturers, and already in the USA more ITE aids are sold than any other type. Again because of their size, the power of these aids is limited when compared to, say, a bodyworn aid, but cosmetically they have found great favour. Some claim that because the microphone of the aid is sited more closely to the natural point of entry of sound to the ear, high frequencies are enhanced and that it is also easier to locate the source of a sound, which in turn may help to counteract the interfering effect of noise. Because they are so small their external controls may be difficult to operate, but some manufacturers have overcome this by having a separate infra-red control box, in principle not unlike the remote infra-red controllers we use with modern TV sets. These aids are necessarily expensive since they have to be 'tailor-made' for each individual, but in due course costs will fall as manufacturing processes become more streamlined. We have little experience as yet of the use of these aids by children. Those trials which have been carried out have suggested that they can used successfully by some children with moderate to severe losses. It is unlikely that this type of aid will be recommended for use with young children because of the problem of growing ears and the difficulty of obtaining a good acoustic seal with the ear.

BONE CONDUCTOR AIDS

The aids which we have discussed up to now all feed sound through an earmould into the ear canal. However, for some children this may not always be possible—their ears may be too deformed to support a mould, there may be no ear canal present, or chronic ear disease may plague the child with frequently discharging ears, which would make the use of an earmould ill-advised. In these circumstances it is possible to fit the child with a bone conductor aid (see Plate VII). When a person hears normally, some sound sets the bones of the skull into vibration. When this happens the inner ear is stimulated directly, responding to sounds which in part bypass the outer and middle ear. You can demonstrate this phenomenon for yourself quite easily by blocking your ears with your thumbs to shut out sound, and tapping or scratching your teeth with your fingernails. You will hear the sounds quite clearly. Bone conductor aids make use of this effect by transferring sound energy directly to the bones of the skull through a special bone vibrator. This is a small device which fits onto the mastoid bone behind the ear and is held in place by a sprung headband. The vibrator can be connected to either a special post-aural aid or a bodyworn aid. Bone conduction aids are very helpful for children who do not have a great sensori-neural loss. Where this is the case, it is difficult to transfer enough power to the cochlea to overcome the loss. The quality of sound provided by bone conductor aids is not as good as that of more conventional receivers nor are they as powerful, so for this reason it is always preferable to use an air conduction aid where this is possible. It is also sometimes difficult to keep the bone conductor correctly placed on the mastoid bone, although decorated headbands combined with hairstyles can often be used imaginatively in the case of girls. Boys with short haircuts present more of a problem. Another problem is the amount of flesh covering the mastoid bone. The thicker and softer the flesh, the more inefficient the transfer of sound energy becomes. For this reason, where the condition which created the need for a bone conductor aid is permanent, it is possible for a small titanium stud to be implanted into the mastoid bone, projecting through the skin. A bone vibrator can now be fixed directly onto the stud. This greatly improves the transfer of energy, and of course there is no problem of holding it in place. Fortunately, the number of children who need to use bone conductor aids is very small and most teachers in ordinary classrooms will not come across them.

Aids Which Use Headphones

Children use a number of other types of hearing aids apart from their personal aids. Of great importance for those children with significant sensori-neural losses are those aids which make use of headphones. There are two main types of these: group hearing aids and speech training units. Necessarily, these aids are considerably larger than personal hearing aids, but this gives them the advantage of producing better sound quality which in itself is enough to justify their use despite their size. Although the maximum gain or the maximum output of these aids is often no greater than that of the most powerful personal aids, the frequency response and freedom from distortion is much better. The frequency response is superior in both the low frequencies and the high. This is often enough to make audible certain of the sounds of speech which cannot be heard through personal aids. It is also possible, due to the high input levels which can be used, to avoid some of the problems of acoustic feedback.

GROUP HEARING AIDS

These are used by groups of hearing impaired children. They are normally found in special schools and in some units, and are either hard-wired into fixed positions or come in the form of a large trolley aid. They are usually mains powered. All the children wear a headset, and have their own microphone so that they can hear their own voices and make their voices heard to others. So all the pupils using the aid are interconnected (see Plate VIII). The teacher also has a microphone and this is connected to the amplifier of the system either by a lead or by a wireless link. Because the teacher is able to talk directly into the microphone, the children receive a very good pattern of what is being said. The effect of background noise is also minimised. Group hearing aids are particularly useful where talking, either by the teacher or by the children themselves or by both, is a prominent feature of the lesson. Properly used, the group hearing aid gives the best possible acoustic information where groups of people are talking together. The controls on these aids are also more accurate than those on personal hearing aids, so it is possible to set the aid to the best possible setting each time it is used.

SPEECH TRAINING UNITS

These aids are very similar to group hearing aids, they have the same excellent acoustic qualities, but they are meant for individual use (see Plate IX). They are really like a single module taken from a group hearing aid, and in fact some group hearing aids simply consist of the same units linked together. They are also, of course, much smaller, are readily portable and are frequently battery powered. This means that they can be carried for use in odd quiet corners or even outside. They are also widely used in the home with very young children. They are particularly useful for conversation work, reading aloud and individual work generally. The child hears his own voice well, and his teacher's voice well in quiet listening conditions. Even if they are used for only a quarter of an hour a day, the acoustic experience they provide is invaluable to the hearing impaired child. Once a child's required settings have been found, they are easy to use, reliable and seldom break down.

Radio Hearing Aids

Personal hearing aids become less effective as the distance from the speaker increases and as the level of background noise rises. Radio hearing aids are designed to overcome these problems. They are therefore essential pieces of equipment for children who are integrating into ordinary classrooms, or any environment regularly visited where background noise levels are relatively high, if full benefit is to be derived from amplification. The actual sound quality of radio aids is no better than that of personal aids but, because the speaker uses a microphone close to the mouth, interference caused by background noise is greatly reduced. This aspect is discussed in more detail in Chapter 7.

All radio aids include two basic parts: a radio transmitter worn by the teacher or parent, and a radio receiver worn by the child. The transmitter has a microphone connected to it and this is used close to the speaker's mouth. The receiver is worn in a convenient place by the child. In use the transmitter sends an FM radio signal to the receiver as the user speaks. It is not unlike a specialised form of 'walkie talkie', except that the child does not have a transmitter and so cannot send radio signals back. Since radio aids are relatively heavy on power, they need to accommodate fairly large batteries and so are quite bulky when compared to personal aids. It is also normal for them to use rechargeable batteries since battery life is no more than a normal working day. Batteries therefore need to be recharged every night if an aid has been used during the day. This applies both to the transmitter and to the receiver.

Radio aids operate using a range of pre-determined radio frequencies specified by the Home Office. Twenty-five such frequencies have been allocated ranging from 171.100 MHz to 175.020 MHz. The radio frequency required is selected by fitting a special crystal oscillator. This can either be built-in, or it can be in the form of a module that the user is able to change, there being a different module for each frequency. It is of course essential for both the transmitter and the receiver to be tuned to the same frequency for the system to work. Some radio receivers are provided with two frequencies, one built-in, and one an interchangeable module, with the facility to switch between the two. Where the user does switch between frequencies, it is of course necessary for a transmitter which transmits on the new frequency to be used. This facility is very useful in ordinary schools where a number of radio frequencies may be in use by several individual children, since it is possible for them all to have radio receivers with a common built-in frequency. They can then switch to this common frequency when they come together as a group—in school assemblies for example.

There are two basic types of radio aid system, known to teachers of the deaf as Type I and Type II.

TYPE I SYSTEMS
These radio systems have a personal hearing aid (or, often now, the equivalent of two) built into them, enabling the aid to be used either as part of a radio system or as a conventional bodyworn aid. The sound is delivered into a button receiver similar to that used by a bodyworn aid, fitting into the earmould in the same way, and attached by a lead to the amplifier, which is in the same box as the radio receiver (see Plate X). The child uses the aid as his personal aid for most of the day, using it as a radio receiver when this is

needed. The sound quality of these systems is good, since they have the same advantages as bodyworn aids of using relatively large button receivers, one for each ear, to deliver the sound. This in turn means that there can be more undistorted low frequency sound, which we know benefits those with greater degrees of hearing loss. Type I systems tend to be larger and heavier than modern bodyworn hearing aids, partly because they have more components in them, partly because they need a larger capacity battery to drive them. For this reason they should be used with a special harness so that they can be held properly in place. All hearing impaired children need to be able to hear the sound of their own voices when they talk. To be able to do this effectively the microphone of the aid which they are using needs to be fairly close to their mouths. The need to wear these aids high on the chest may sometimes be avoided where a small lapel-type microphone, pinned to the child's clothing, can be used. The only problem with this is that an extra lead has to be accommodated. However, most teachers and parents prefer this option where it is available.

TYPE II SYSTEMS
These systems simply comprise a transmitter and radio receiver. They do not have a personal aid built in. This means that they can only be used with another amplifying device such as a personal aid—the radio receiver captures the transmitted signal and the hearing aid amplifies it (see Plate XI). Type II systems can be used with both post-aural and bodyworn personal aids, though their use is far more common with the former. The advantage of a Type II system is that it can be used with the personal aid which the child is used to wearing all the time and usually this means consistency of sound. Since the power for the amplification of the signal is provided by the battery of the personal hearing aid, battery size and capacity is not so much of a problem, but nevertheless batteries need to be recharged each night. Also, with some Type II systems which are in use all day long, it has been found necessary to change batteries at lunchtime to ensure full operation up to the end of the school day. Some

Type II systems have a microphone built into the radio receiver so that the child can hear his own voice, but most rely on the microphone of the personal aid to perform this function. There is little difference between the transmitters of Type I and Type II systems and in theory, provided the radio frequencies are matched they can be used with either type. It is also possible for a Type I system to be used as a Type II system, but we would not recommend this since they were not designed for that purpose.

There are two ways by which the radio receiver can deliver its signal to the personal hearing aid for amplification—by a direct electrical link, or by magnetic induction. Of these two, the former is without doubt the better as far as sound quality is concerned. By this method a special lead connects the radio receiver to the personal aid. The personal aid needs to be fitted with a direct audio input specifically for this purpose. Nowadays most post-aural aids which have an audio input use a special 'shoe' to connect the lead to the hearing aid contacts. This makes it much more convenient to connect and disconnect the lead. It also means that for many aids the same type of lead can be used, since the shoe connector effectively converts the great variety of contact configurations in use into a standard format. Once one has the appropriate shoe, it is of course much easier to obtain a standard lead than one which is tailor made for a particular model of aid. Most commercially available post-aural hearing aids are now fitted with a direct audio input facility. Unfortunately at the time of writing this does not apply to National Health Service aids, none of which are fitted with direct audio input. This means that children who need to use radio aids will have to be provided with commercial aids, but fortunately current regulations allow such special provision for children to be made through the NHS.

Unlike post-aural aids there are very few bodyworn aids that have a direct audio input, although those that do have been used very successfully with hearing impaired children. Occasionally, there have been one or two difficulties with connecting leads in some combinations. It is not difficult to obtain a lead to connect a Type II radio receiver to one bodyworn aid, but sometimes it is necessary to have leads specially made up where the child wears two bodyworn aids—and most will. Another problem which sometimes occurs is that the radio signal can be rather weak, and this results in a background 'shushing' noise making itself heard. This is usually due to the fact that the lead which connects the radio receiver to an aid often doubles as the aerial to the radio signal from the transmitter. If a post-aural aid is used there is no problem with this, because the lead up to the ear is quite long and is more or less vertical. With a bodyworn aid the distance covered by the lead is much shorter and it is often horizontal, so the signal the aerial receives is not as strong. Where this occurs the only solution is to try to arrange the leads so that this does not happen, or to try different radio receivers. If the problem still cannot be resolved, and the power of a bodyworn aid is needed, the only answer may be to use a Type I system instead.

The second way by which the signal can be transferred to personal aids is magnetic induction. Many personal hearing aids, including National Health aids, have a special coil of wire called an inductance coil (or telecoil) fitted inside them. This was originally designed for use with telephone receivers and inductance loop systems, which are still used today. The basic principal involved is that of the electrical transformer. The signal is fed into a coil (or loop) of wire (the primary) and this generates a changing magnetic field which mirrors the variations of the input sound. If the coil fitted in the hearing aid (the secondary) is within this changing magnetic field an electrical current is induced into the coil, and this can then be amplified by the hearing aid and converted back into sound. Type II radio aid systems can use this process, by routing the signal from the receiver into a coil of wire worn around the neck, called a neckloop. The child's personal post-aural aids are then switched to the telecoil position and the aid is then energised by the changing magnetic field of the neckloop. Neckloops are favoured by some teachers because they are easy for children to take on and off. Many teenagers are said to prefer them also, though in our experience this is far from being a universal response. The great disadvantage of neckloops is that the quality of sound that they produce is not as good nor as consistent as that provided by direct inputs. They are therefore not really suitable for children with anything other than a moderate loss, and even these would in our view benefit more from the use of a direct input. Another effect which can be annoying to the wearer is that the strength of the electromagnetic signal can vary as the head is moved and the angle of the telecoil in the post-aural aid changes in relation to the neckloop. Bodyworn hearing aids are also usually fitted with telecoils and although attempts have been made to use Type II systems and magnetic inductance with such aids this has not proved to be successful. It is unlikely that a child who is sufficiently hearing impaired to need the power of a bodyworn aid would benefit from such an approach; only direct input could provide the quality of signal necessary. When magnetic inductance is used with radio aids in this way, the telecoil in the personal hearing aid has to be switched into circuit. When this is done, sometimes, the microphone in the aid is switched off. This means that the wearer cannot hear their own voice. In these circumstances it is necessary to use a radio receiver which has an environmental microphone built in. The signal from the wearer's voice is now fed into the neckloop together with the incoming radio signal. Some ear-level aids with direct audio input facility do not have a telecoil and yet people lacking in knowledge are fitting children with these aids with neckloops. Such children will receive *none* of the signal from the radio transmitter.

While radio hearing aid systems are of great benefit to children, they do have some drawbacks. Their potential is best realised when individual children are integrating into ordinary classrooms. They are not so useful where groups of hearing impaired children are involved, in special schools for example, since there is no means for them to hear each other, except through the environmental microphones of their aids. In these circumstances they offer no advantage over personal aids, except that the teacher's voice will be clearer. So activities such as group discussions, or those where the children are expected to make frequent spoken contributions to a lesson are better served by the use of a group hearing aid.

Radio hearing aids have also been found to be of great help in the home with young children, particularly once they have reached the toddler stage. But such use falls outside the scope of this book and is well dealt with elsewhere.[2]

Infra-Red Systems

Occasionally the use of an infra-red system may be suggested to teachers or parents. In use they are very similar to FM radio systems, except instead of using radio frequencies to transmit the signal, this is carried by a beam of infra-red light (see Plate XII). The speaker wears a transmitter and the child wears a receiver, but these must not be covered by clothing. It can be used as either a Type I or a Type II system. Where it is used as a Type II system the signal can either be fed into a direct audio input, or a neckloop can be used. Because the light emitted from the transmitter cannot pass through walls, unlike FM radio systems, the signal is confined to the room in which it is being used. This can sometimes be an advantage. However, since the system relies on the light being reflected off the walls and ceiling, the use of infra-red systems is much less effective out of doors. Also in halls and large rooms the strength of the reflected light may not be strong enough to provide a good signal. However, it is possible to overcome this problem in halls which are used regularly by installing special secondary transmitters called transponders. Sometimes strong sunshine streaming through windows can have an effect and the fitting of blinds may be necessary in some classrooms where this occurs. Infra-red systems are worth considering in circumstances where it is difficult to use FM radio systems, for example in large schools where all the available radio frequencies have been used up by individually integrating hearing impaired children or where a particular school site is subject to frequent radio interference.

Cochlear Implants

Although cochlear implantation is a surgical procedure, the cochlear implant is simply another type of hearing aid designed to deliver a sound signal to the brain of the user. However, our experience of use of cochlear implants with children in this country is so limited that it is not possible here to add to the comments we have already made on this subject in Chapter 1.

SELECTING AIDS FOR CHILDREN

The selection of an appropriate personal hearing aid for a young child, especially one with a congenital sensori-neural hearing loss, is a matter for skilled judgment. Clearly the most important factors influencing the choice will be the type, cause and degree of hearing loss that a child has. In the early days this may simply involve selecting an instrument of an appropriate level of power. It is important that the aid should have sufficient power, but also that it should not be too powerful for a particular loss. Then other factors need to be taken into account: What is the age of the child? Will a post-aural aid or a bodyworn aid be easier for parents to manage? Will a radio aid be used? Will spare parts be readily available? Can the aid be easily repaired? Are teachers more familiar with one make of aid or another? And so on. There are so many personal hearing aids available that there is some sense in the relevant authorities attempting to standardise on a narrow range of models so that some consistency can be maintained. It is also well worth bearing in mind that most of the recent developments in hearing aid design have been in making aids smaller, or in controlling the sounds delivered to the user in more sophisticated ways. They have not actually led to a better overall frequency response or an increase in undistorted gain and output. These features are largely determined by the microphones and receivers used in hearing aids, and there only a limited number of different types of these available. Since most hearing aid manufacturers buy-in these components from the same few suppliers, they have to design their aids within the same constraints. It is also important to appreciate that it may well be necessary to change the type of hearing aid issued to a child as circumstances change or as we learn more about the child's residual hearing capacity.

DETERMINING AMPLIFICATION NEEDS

Once a particular aid has been chosen for a child, it is then necessary to set the aid to an appropriate level for that child, to select the frequency response and possibly incorporate some output limitation. Again this is a job for an audiologist, but the observations of teachers and parents of how well they think a child is using the aid are of vital importance, since the process is an ongoing one. If the aid and the settings are appropriate, the volume control of the hearing aid should not need to be turned beyond about half to two-thirds of its travel. This is to ensure that there is sufficient reserve power to cope with different listening environments. If you find that a child seems to manage better with the volume of the aid turned up higher than this in normal listening conditions, then it would be wise to ask for a hearing-aid review. Many profoundly hearing impaired children wearing high-power aids may, however, need to set the volume control close to maximum.

There are two principal ways by which audiologists determine amplification needs. The first is by using what is called a 'prescriptive' method, the second is by giving the hearing-aid user a series of listening tests. There are a number of prescriptive methods in use, but they all work on the similar principle of applying one of a number of formulae to the known hearing status of an individual. Usually the formula selected is applied to the results of pure tone threshold tests (where the person being tested responds to the quietest levels of certain frequencies which they can just hear), since these yield some of the most reliable and repeatable results. The aim is to use this approach to get the amplification requirements approximately right and then to 'fine-tune' the aid as the result of further listening tests. Most of the prescriptive methods have been originated with deafened adults in mind and very few have been specifically for children with a congenital hearing loss. One such method developed by the authors is extremely simple and yet has proved to be very effective. One simply takes the child's pure tone hearing loss at the three frequencies 250Hz, 500Hz and 2kHz, adds the values together, divides this total by six and then adds 80. The figure which results is the level at which the child needs to listen to speech, and is the level to which the output of the aid should be set. So, for example, if a child's hearing loss shown on the pure tone audiogram for the three frequencies indicated above is 80dB(HL), 90dB(HL) and 100dB(HL), then the output required is (80+90+100)/6 + 80 = 125dB(SPL). This method works much better than those developed for adults.

However, all prescriptive methods have their limitations; they are simply estimates of the amplification levels needed by a child. The optimum levels can only be found following a series of tests which require the child to discriminate speech in a range of listening conditions. These 'speech tests of hearing', as they are called, are both involved and time-consuming. They need to be carried out by specialists, but as soon as a child is able to perform satisfactorily on such tests he should be given the opportunity to undergo them. Properly executed, such tests provide the most accurate information about the type of amplification a child should be given to enable discrimination of the sounds of spoken language most easily.

Another popular way of attempting to estimate whether a particular hearing aid or its setting is appropriate is by carrying out 'aided threshold testing'. Having completed a threshold test for pure tones either listening through headphones or to loudspeakers, the child then listens through the hearing aids to the same range of sounds (usually slightly modified pure tones), presented by loudspeakers. By comparing the two results it is possible to determine how much amplification the child is getting from the aids at that particular setting. This is useful information, and certainly indicates when an aid is not suitable. It reveals what proportion of the spectrum of speech sounds the child should be able to hear, but it does not tell you how to set the aid so that speech can most easily be discriminated. The findings still need to be supplemented by properly conducted speech tests of hearing. Aided thresholds need to be carried out with special equipment in specially treated rooms, and the test procedure is as yet not well standardised. However, in the right circumstances it is quick and easy to administer.

MAINTAINING HEARING AIDS

If hearing aids are to be used effectively by children and their teachers, it is important that they are maintained properly. Since personal aids are those which get the most use, they are often the ones which go wrong first and which need the most amount of attention. The checking of the more specialist type of aids, such as headphone aids and radio hearing aids, demands a higher level of skill and other than simple listening tests these are best left to teachers of the deaf to check. So we will concentrate here on the checking and maintenance of personal aids.

Visual Checks

The child's aid should be examined for any signs of damage (e.g., cracked case, broken switches). Sound should be able to freely pass into the microphone, no foreign bodies such as food or dirt should be obstructing this pathway. All controls should be checked and reset if they have been disturbed. The receiver on a bodyworn aid should be checked to ensure that it is the correct one for the child. It can easily be 'exchanged' accidentally in a playground melée.

Earmould Checks

Careful checks should be made of the earmoulds. They should be cleaned each evening with a little warm soapy water and a toothbrush (spare one!) or pipe cleaner. Hopefully this will prevent the build-up of wax within the sound tubes. Blow through the tubing so as to ensure that the sound tube is completely free of condensation and debris. It is possible to obtain a special air puffer to do this job, and teachers with a number of hearing impaired children in their care may find this useful.

Battery Checks

This in our view involves two aspects. First, the daily 'is it making the aid work?' check which is carried out as follows:

1   Switch aid on.
2   (i)   For a pocket aid, turn the volume to full and hold the receiver a lead length from the microphone. The aid should produce a characteristic squeal of acoustic feedback.
    (ii) For a post-aural aid turn on the aid to full volume and direct the plastic elbow towards the ear canal—the aid should squeal.

3   If the expected results in 2, above, do not occur then the battery should be replaced and the procedure repeated.

4   Parents and teachers should be provided with a listening device called a *stetoclip*, which is used in a similar manner to a doctors stethoscope except that, instead of listening to the patients heart, one listens to the quality of sound being reproduced by the hearing aid. Parent or teacher should become accustomed to the power of the aid and know a volume at which it is comfortable to listen. (Special acoustic attenuators are available which, when fitted, prevent sounds which are too loud for a normally hearing person from reaching the ear. With one of these it is possible to listen to an aid at the setting a child uses, so that one can listen more realistically for distortion, which usually only occurs when the aid is set to a high volume. If an attenuator is used then the aid can be listened to at full power, but *not* otherwise.) The listener should then listen through the aid and check for low power or distorted output. If the battery is suspected to be the cause of the fault then it should be replaced.

The second aspect of an approach to hearing-aid power supply is the battery changing guideline (see Table I). This approach was pioneered by us and we believe that for the busy teacher, especially with young children, this is the most practical approach to ensuring that the child's aid is working at full strength. We and former research students have calculated the service life in hours of a large variety of hearing aid/battery combinations and have suggested 'safe' change times (Shaw, reported in *Educational Audiology*[1]).

Mainstream teachers should be aware that the penlight cells used in body hearing aids decay over time, so the child would gradually receive less and less through the aid whereas the 'button cells' used in post-aural aids cut out quite suddenly.

If the teacher speaks into the microphone it is possible to check the quality of sound being produced and whether there are high levels of 'aid noise'. This is the background 'shush' from the aid when there is no input to the microphone.

If all appears well after the above tests then the aid can be fitted to the child. With bodyworn aids it is desirable that a well-fitting harness is used and that the connecting leads are tucked carefully out of the child's reach. The aids can then be set to an appropriate level and switched on. Mainstream teachers should be told what all these settings are and it should be recorded in the child's records in the classroom. At the setting designated by the specialist teacher of the deaf or educational audiologist it should be possible to deliver the necessary amplification to the child without acoustic feedback. We cannot stress too highly the need for correctly fitting earmoulds and, of course, a prime test of this is whether they can deliver the levels of amplification required, without acoustic feedback occurring.

When there is failure of the aid it should be possible for a mainstream teacher, who has a supply of spares and has had a modest amount of training, to test by substitution and effect a repair. It would be even better if each child had with him in the classroom a spare aid, and then the class teacher would not need to interrupt classroom work but could look at the

Table 1
Battery changing guidelines

Make and Model	CP1	CP101	CP6
BE10 Series (11, 12, 14 & 16)	Every two weeks (165h)	Every four weeks (347h)	–
BE30 Series (31 & 32)	Every week (estimated)	Every two weeks (178h)	–
BE50 Series (51)	Twice a week (40h)	Twice a week (66h)	–
Danavox 775PP	Twice a week (62h)	Once a week (84h)	–
Oticon E22P	Twice a week (47h)	Twice a week (69h)	–
Phonak PPCL	Twice a week (47h)	Twice a week (71h)	–
Philips 8276	Twice a week (51h)	Once a week (89h)	–
Unitron E1P	Twice a week (estimated)	Once a week (96h)	–
BW61	–	–	Once a week (129h)
BW81	–	–	Twice a week (71h)
Philips 8146	–	–	Twice a week (55h)
Windsor	–	–	Twice a week (52h)

broken aid later. A step-by-step approach such as that described below can be very helpful to teachers inexperienced in handling hearing aids:

1   Examine the aid and check that it is switched on and that M (Microphone) is selected.
2   Ensure that the earmoulds are not blocked with wax.
3   Shake the aid to see if any components have become loose internally. If so, then it is likely that specialist assistance will be required. It is still worth proceeding with the sequence since the loose component may not be responsible for the fault.
4   Ensure that the battery is in correctly and not upside down as sometimes happens.
5   Ensure that the plastic elbow of a post-aural aid is free from blockage.

If the problem still persists proceed to:

6   Replace the battery and recheck the aid.
7   Replace the lead on the pocket aids and recheck the aid.
8   Replace the receiver on pocket aids and recheck the aid.

It is a good idea to leave replacement parts in the aid when moving through the checks since dual faults do occur and could be missed. If the checks and substitutions above do not cure the problem, then the aid must be replaced. Any mainstream teacher with a hearing impaired child in the class should be able to telephone for assistance in such cases, since it would be educationally disastrous to leave a deaf child in a mainstream class without amplification.

Checks such as those described above do help to speed up the repairs of aids for children since it is not uncommon for aids to be returned to the manufacturer with no other problem than a flat battery or faulty connecting lead.

The peripatetic teacher of the deaf should ensure that:

1   Mainstream teachers have a month's supply of batteries.
2   A stetoclip.
3   Mainstream teachers know how to check for battery problems and replace the batteries.

The above checks can all be carried out by trained parents or mainstream teachers but the peripatetic teacher should also carry out electro-acoustic tests using specialised equipment such as the hearing-aid test box. Only then is it possible to be sure that the hearing aid meets the manufacturer's specifications. We believe that such tests should be carried out at least monthly, to supplement the daily checks outlined above.

Testing Hearing Aids Using Electro-Acoustic Methods

HAND-HELD TESTER

This is a cheap and relatively simple-to-operate piece of equipment which can be used by a peripatetic teacher to check all types of hearing aids except varieties requiring headphones. It consists of a special coupler attached to a sound-level meter which measures the sound pressure level generated in a specially designed cavity by a particular aid (see Plate XIII). Its main purpose is to check the output of hearing aids and the field strength of the electromagnetic loop induction systems (e.g. loops in classrooms). The aid check is made in a close-to-real-world situation in that—with a bodyworn hearing aid for example—the child would wear the aid, the earphone receiver being taken from his ear and connected to the ear simulator of the test machine (a 2c.c. coupler). The unit provides a readout of the sound pressure developed in the simulator. It covers the complete range of sound pressure delivered by hearing aids. Teachers will usually use a speech input signal so that an approximate idea of the amplified speech level being directed to the child could be obtained. The class teacher would be guided as to the required volume setting for a young child. By routine testing of the aid at the user-setting, it soon becomes obvious if deterioration in output has occurred for a speech input signal.

THE HEARING AID TEST BOX

A hearing-aid test box is an instrument which enables the electro-acoustic characteristics of a hearing aid to be measured accurately. There is a range of such instruments, varying from highly sophisticated and expensive laboratory instruments, to more basic portable devices. Even the latter are quite expensive, costing in the region of £4,000 at the time of writing. But it is a false economy for an authority to have tens of thousands of pounds worth of amplification equipment in use by children and not have the means to be able to check regularly that it is working properly and doing what it is supposed to do. All test boxes have three essential parts: a sound generator, a carefully designed acoustic chamber, and a measurement system. The sound generator produces sounds which can be accurately controlled by the operator in terms of their frequency and intensity; the acoustic chamber provides a controlled environment in which the sounds can be made; and the measuring circuit measures the sound emerging from the receiver of the hearing aid. In operation, the microphone of the hearing aid is positioned accurately in the acoustic chamber, a series of sounds are fed into the microphone of the aid under test, and a special coupler, linked to the measuring circuit, is attached to the receiver of the hearing aid. The parameters of the sounds going into the microphone of the aid are displayed, as are the values of the sound coming out of the receiver. The two can now be compared. It is normal for a range of frequencies to be tested. Modern test boxes are microprocessor controlled and can be completely automatic in operation. Results are displayed on a small screen or display panel, and usually a printout of the results can be made. The printout may either be in the form of a graph or a table of numbers, whichever is more convenient for the task in hand. The whole process takes about two minutes per aid.

It is the responsibility of those specialists (audiologists and teachers of the deaf) working with hearing impaired children to ensure that the hearing aids always meet the design criteria and in order to achieve this the aids must be frequently tested in a standardised fashion in a hearing-aid test box. Hearing-aid manufacturers produce comprehensive data sheets on each hearing aid measured to British, International and American

Standards (BSI, IEC, and ANSI) and it is against these standards that the aids must be measured. It is worth noting that manufacturers normally produce their data on quite a large sample of hearing aids so their results are averages. What you measure on a single hearing aid may vary slightly, but the tolerances are narrow and should be no wider than 5dB.

The development of the portable test box was a very important innovation as far as ensuring the efficient day-to-day use of hearing aids by children is concerned (see Plate XIV). In our view, peripatetic teachers visiting homes and advising in mainstream schools should have a portable test box available. In this way we believe that hearing aids will be much more frequently tested than if they were taken for testing to a clinic. This book is not the place for detailed descriptions of how to use the test box (these can be seen in *Educational Audiology*[1]), but readers may well be interested in what measures we think should be made on hearing aids and recorded for subsequent comparison:

1　Maximum gain
2　Maximum gain at 1000Hz
3　Maximum output
4　Maximum output at 1000Hz
5　Basic frequency response
6　Harmonic distortion
7　Random noise
8　Frequency response at normal user setting
9　Harmonic distortion at normal user setting

Maximum gain.　The input to the aid is set to 50dB(SPL) or 60dB(SPL) and the output is measured across the frequencies with the volume control on maximum. The frequency where the output is greatest should be noted, together with the value of this output and also the output at 1000Hz. The input value should then be subtracted from these values to give maximum gain and maximum gain at 1000Hz.

Maximum output. The procedure is the same as above except that the input selected is 90dB(SPL) to drive the aid into saturation. The greatest value of the output at any frequency, together with the maximum output at 1000Hz, is recorded.

Basic frequency response. Different standards measure the frequency response of an aid in slightly different ways. The volume control of the aid is adjusted to a particular level depending on the method being used. This is sometimes called the 'reference test gain control setting'. A commonly used method is to select an input of 60dB(SPL) and then adjust the volume control of the aid until at 1000Hz the output sound pressure is 100dB(SPL). The output is then measured across the range of frequencies at that volume control setting to give the basic frequency response.

Harmonic distortion. This is perhaps the most difficult parameter to quantify by simple listening tests and yet it is most important if the sound delivered to the child is not to be unacceptably distorted. The child's aid should be set to the level used for the measurement of the frequency response and the input set to 70dB SPL. Total harmonic distortion should be measured at 500, 800 and 1600Hz (these frequencies will be a function of the test box in use). Distortion should not exceed 10 per cent.

Random noise. Hearing-aids generate random electronic noise as well as amplifying sounds that we want. It is important that this random noise does not reach a level which would obscure the signals we wish the child to hear. One way to test for this is to place the hearing-aid in the test box and with an input of 60dB SPL at 1000Hz adjust the gain so that the coupler output is 100dB(SPL) (so that the gain equals 40dB—the setting sometimes used for the basic frequency response). The frequency response is then recorded. The sound source should then be switched off. The noise–sound pressure level in the test chamber should now be negligible. The total sound pressure level in the coupler is now measured and this should be at least 30dB below the basic frequency response curve.

As well as checks which relate to the specification 'quality control' we believe that the teacher should also test the aid at a pupil's usual setting. We also think it is very valuable to use the 'in the ear' adaptor, if one is available, to check the aid's response whilst it is still attached to the pupil's earmould. In particular, this approach will bring to light the use of very narrow earmould tubing, or narrow bore diameter, features which greatly reduce the passage of high frequencies, which are vital for speech discrimination. In post-aural earmoulds a chemical reaction between the tubing and the mould results in the tube shrinking and becoming hard. This effectively strangles the signal. Routine testing through the mould should discover this problem. If test box facilities are not available we would strongly recommend changing the tubing at least every month, and definitely if it is starting to become discoloured.

It is important that the tests are carried out in quiet conditions. Test boxes are not soundproof and high levels of ambient will affect the results. This is particularly true for distortion and random noise measurements. If there is a sudden increase in noise whilst one of the measurements is being made, that measurement should be repeated as soon as the noise has subsided.

This may sound a complicated routine, but with only a little familiarity test boxes are quick and easy to use. It does not take long to learn how to use them. In many establishments the testing is carried out by classroom assistants, and in some by the children themselves. Parents have been trained to use them too. The wider availability of hearing-aid test boxes will undoubtedly bring about great improvements in the efficiency and consistency of hearing-aid use by hearing impaired children.

References
1 Tucker, I. and Nolan, M., *Educational Audiology*. Croom Helm, 1986.
2 Nolan, M. and Tucker, I., *The Hearing Impaired Child and the Family*, 2nd edn, Souvenir Press Ltd, 1988.

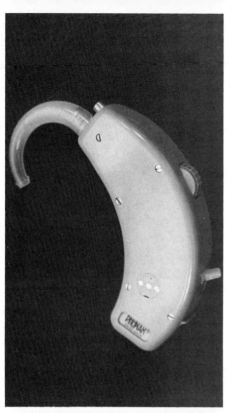

V *Left:* A) An ear-level aid.
Below: B) A 'mini' and a 'standard' ear-level aid.

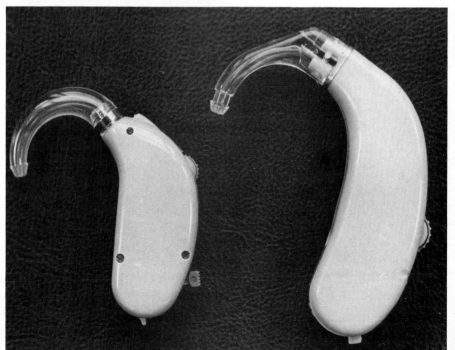

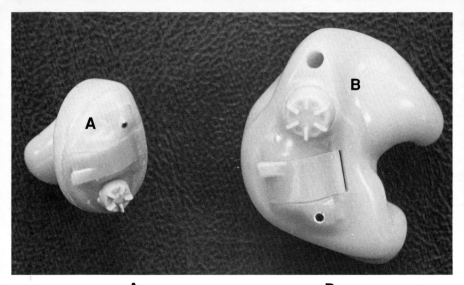

VI In the ear (ITE) aids. *Left:* A) Canal aid. *Right:* B) Standard in the ear aid.

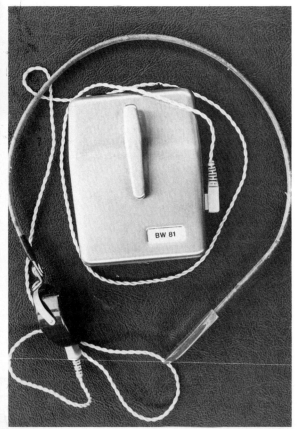

VII A bone conductor aid.

3 Communication Approaches Used in the Education of Hearing Impaired Children

There is one simple statement which can be made about the communication approaches used in the education of deaf children—that it is a highly complex question! Indeed were this not the case it would have been resolved years ago, rather than rumbling on through the centuries as it has. New evidence, new practices frequently serve to cloud issues rather than clarify them. Hearing parents of newly diagnosed deaf children particularly, are often thrown into a maelstrom of conflicting ideologies, and yet ultimately, in spite of their limited knowledge and experience of deafness in children, it is they who will need to reach the difficult decisions which will affect their offspring for the whole of their lives. Hard though this responsibility may be to bear, it is infinitely preferable to a return to the days when parents were given little say by professionals in what was best for their child. However, in order to exercise their responsibilities parents need information, and this chapter attempts to provide some of that information.

LANGUAGE AND COMMUNICATION

It is perhaps worth making the point from the outset, that language and communication are not the same thing. Language is a conventional system by means of which ideas are deliberately communicated. It has a structure and a vocabulary, governed by certain rules which are followed by those who use that language. Different languages have different rules. But it is possible to communicate without using language—the look, the touch, the gesture which in a given situation conveys a thought to others. The communication which occurs may or may not be intended, but it is difficult to transfer that thought to a wider audience unless it is re-expressed in a more structured way—a way which uses rules which that audience knows. Basically, communication is about passing a message, whereas language is about passing a message in a conventional, systematic way to others who use the system. So children, be they hearing or deaf, are able to communicate long before they are able to use language for that purpose. The advantage of using a language, of course, is that it is able to convey more ideas, and ideas of greater complexity, more quickly, more efficiently to more people.

The communication approaches used with deaf children, therefore, are intended not simply to allow communication to occur, but to bring about the acquisition of language. The goal is to ensure that every deaf child has a secure first language, be that spoken or signed. It is also worth mentioning here that the way in which a first language is *acquired* is quite different to the process by which a second language is normally *learned*. Some recent techniques for second language teaching however are modelled on first language acquisition, and by like token some ways of trying to teach language to deaf children incorporate second language teaching methods. We use the term 'first language' in place of the more usual 'mother tongue', since the latter suggests talking and this may not be appropriate for some deaf children.

There is a fundamental division in the communication approaches used by parents and teachers with deaf children: those which rely primarily on hearing and talking, and those which incorporate, or are mainly composed of, manual elements. This means a basic difference in the manner in which the auditory and visual channels are used. Readers may be aware that the sense of hearing is particularly good at analysing time sequences, whilst vision handles spatial information well. The biological difference between the two modalities to some extent determines the form of a language which uses the ear for its reception and that of a language received by the eye.

AUDITORY APPROACHES

Auditory approaches are sometimes referred to as the 'oral method' or 'oralism', but these are terms which mask basic and very important differences between the different types. The 'oral method' really refers to a system which is perhaps better called *traditional oralism*. It is rooted in history and was in use long before it was thought possible or beneficial to amplify sounds for deaf children. Consequently, it placed great emphasis on lip-reading and developing the skill of the visual channel to interpret spoken information. It has lasted well into this century and indeed it was still practised by some teachers until quite recently. The emphasis was on watching rather than on listening. But more important was the way in which traditional oralists believed that language could best be taught to deaf children. The focus was on teaching language, rather than children acquiring language. The techniques used were, as we now know, in complete conflict with the process of language acquisition as we understand it today. Language was taught in a systematic, logical way. It was broken down into its basic elements, and then presented to the child in a seemingly logical order. A group of children progressed to the next step, once they had learned the one being taught. So there would be vocabulary lists to be learned, followed by syntax. 'Why?' questions would not be introduced until 'What?', 'Where?' and 'When?' questions had been tackled. The tenses were taught, present tense first, then the past, then the future. Throughout there was emphasis on the *form* of the language rather its meaning. Language was 'taught' rather than used. The logic was that of the adult, not of the child. There was great stress on repetition and grammatical exercises, most of them mechanical. Writing had a central role to play since this, in the adult's eyes, gave an unambiguous representation of the language which was being taught. Systematic correction of children's mistakes was also considered important. However, children who were able to write pages of grammatical exercises working from books or worksheets with relatively few errors nevertheless had great difficulty in conveying their own thoughts and ideas in continuous writing. Whilst they could cope with a few stilted sentences with simple basic constructions, as soon they tried to move on to more complex ideas, problems arose. Because of the emphasis on lip-reading, speech was often very much slowed with considerable over-articulation, since it was felt that this helped both speech and understanding. Speech correction had a prominent place in the classroom, and a child's spoken contributions to lessons were frequently interrupted to enable him to have a second or third attempt to pronounce a word or phrase in order to render it more intelligible. The whole ethos of traditional oralism was one of highlighting mistakes and attempting to put them right.

A modern development of traditional oralism is *structured oralism*. With the availability of hearing aids, the balance between the visual and auditory aspects of teaching language was changed. Whilst lip-reading is still considered to have an essential place, much greater use of the auditory channel is made. Language is still taught through the planning of structured processes or sequences, and from early stages much attention is still paid to the form of language. There is a systematic intervention in the learning process, be that in relation to spoken language or to writing. Teachers set out to cover certain vocabulary and also language structures, they decide what to teach and in what order. Much of the language content of any lesson is therefore predetermined by the teacher. Systematic correction and repetition still have a place. Sometimes aspects of this approach are encapsulated in a 'language scheme'. A good example of this is the Guidelines English Course developed at the Woodford School by F.J. Thomas which aims to cover all the main structures of English. When it was developed, it was designed principally for use in the primary school, the structures being taught in story form. Children spent about an hour each day on the programme, though presumably the techniques were carried over to other lessons during the day. Structured oral approaches are not without their advantages, not the least being the consistency and the controlled progression which they bring to teaching. Young or inexperienced teachers often find security in the organised approach and are freed to concentrate on how to teach deaf children with the greatest effect in the knowledge that what they are teaching is part of an overall plan.

Another of the approaches which do not incorporate a manual element is the *maternal reflective* approach. Developed in Holland and described by Van Uden,[1] this approach takes as its starting point the acquisition of language by ordinary hearing children, rather than an analysis of adult language. Early childhood conversation and interaction with care- giving adults are key elements on which to focus. In particular it examines how mothers of young hearing children foster language development in their offspring. What are the essential features of the way a mother and her deaf baby converse that promote development? Can we apply this knowledge to the situation of the deaf baby and its mother? Can this then be translated into a viable classroom practice?

Conversation can only take place where the participants talk and listen in turn (although mothers of young babies often have to take the baby's turn as well), and in the classroom the teacher is as much a listener as are the children. The way in which the conversation develops is not pre-determined but it progresses as the ideas flow from the group with all contributions playing a valued part. However, since conversation is fleeting and since many of the deaf children participating will have a less than perfect grasp of the spoken language they are using, the conversation is later written down. This becomes what Van Uden calls a 'deposit' and children and teacher return to this some time afterwards, probably the next day, and reconsider what was said and how it was said. The written word thus has a very important role to play, and it allows children to 'reflect' on the flow of the conversation and in particular upon the structural aspects which might otherwise pass them by. This permanent record of a linguistic experience becomes a valuable resource for developing language. This use of the written word is quite different to that of traditional or structured oralism.

Whilst sharing a similar starting point to the maternal reflective approach *natural auralism* differs in certain important ways. The term 'natural auralism' highlights the two key elements of the approach—that language is expected to be acquired naturally by the child and that the child will do this aurally, i.e. primarily through the auditory channel. It is not an accident that the word 'aural' has replaced 'oral', for the emphasis is first and foremost on listening. As with most other approaches used in the education of deaf children, the seeds of natural auralism can be traced back into the depths of history, but it is only with the relatively recent increase in our knowledge of first language acquisition by babies and young children and the development of modern technology that this approach has evolved into its present form—a form which is now quite different to its early manifestations. The fundamental belief is that all children, including those with hearing losses, acquire their mother tongue by following similar processes, interacting in a conversational way within a family or family-type situation (see Plate XV). It will take longer for deaf children to do this but the ingredients necessary to make it happen will be the same. For teachers to continue the conversational environment of the home at school is far from easy and demands considerable skill and adjustment on their part. The traditional balance between the roles and status of teacher and taught is noticeably different. It is *not* a practice where teacher dominated language is 'poured' over the child in the hope that some of it will stick, but one in which the emergent language of the child, stimulated by his own interests and activities, is shared with the teacher. Unlike traditional oralism, a first language is not something to be taught, but a tool to be used. Natural auralists believe that, where parents are hearing, deaf children have a better chance of acquiring their natural first language through listening, and that means gradually but consistently learning to use what residual hearing remains, so that the necessary listening skills can be fostered. Structured oral approaches and the maternal reflective method stress the need for the use of amplification and residual hearing, but they are not as dependent upon it. Natural auralism means a 'high-tech' approach to the use of amplification, which needs not simply to be provided, but must be the very best, consistently used and subjected to frequent electro-acoustic checking. Whilst the aim is to use residual hearing to the full, this does not mean that the auditory sense will not be supported by the gestural, visual and contextual clues that are part of all linguistic communication, especially where young language-learners are involved. Natural auralism is not a uni-sensory approach. But the part played by the written word is quite different to its use in any of the other forms of oralism. It is not used in a formal way to supplement the experience of spoken language, nor can it be the medium through which language is learned. Rather it is an alternative way of revealing the language a child already possesses.

APPROACHES INCORPORATING MANUAL ELEMENTS

Many of the approaches used with hearing impaired children include a manual component, where the hands are used in a formalised way to support or to convey information to the 'listener'. This formalised component is not to be confused with natural gesture, which is used in all communication particularly with young children, be they hearing or not. The form of the manual components differ greatly, but can broadly be divided into two groups: systems that support or represent English, and those which are separate languages.

Of the systems devised to support English some are intended to make a spoken message more readily intelligible. A typical example of this is *cued speech*. This seeks to clarify spoken language by making lip-reading, or speech-reading as it is more accurately called, easier to follow. Lip-reading is a skill which many deaf children develop quite spontaneously, but it is beset by ambiguities. Many phonemes look very similar on the lips and confusions can occur. Cued speech seeks to minimise these potential confusions. It employs a set of manual cues to do this. The National Cued Speech Association of the USA has recently issued guidelines[2] for the definition of cued speech: 'An accurate description of cued speech must include at least the three basic ideas in the following statement: "Cued speech is a lip-reading support system which (1) utilizes hand configurations (eight in English) in locations (four in English) near the mouth (2) to supplement the normal visual manifestations of speech (3) in such a way as to render the spoken language through vision alone."' The cues thus consist of eight hand configurations, and four hand positions. Only one hand is used. By themselves these hand configurations and positions do not contain enough distinctive information to be comprehensible. They cannot replace the information on the lips, so can only be used in conjunction with lip-reading. The consonants are cued by eight hand shapes, each one signalling a different group. The shapes are arranged so that consonants that look similar on the lips have very different hand shapes, so 't' and 'd' for example, belong to different hand-shape groups. Consonants belonging to the same group and represented by the same hand shape look different on the lips. So 't' and 'm' have the same hand shape. The vowels are represented by four different hand positions relative to the chin. (N.B.: Cues have to be made close to the face so that they are in the same field of view as the lips.) Again the same principle is followed: vowels which look similar to each other are signalled by different hand positions, and those which are clearly different to look at e.g. 'e' as in 'get' and 'u' as in 'blue' share the same hand position. Cued speech was devised by Dr Orin Cornett in 1966. The principle of supporting lip-reading by a signalling system was not new, but cued speech became the most widely used of such systems amongst English language speakers here, in the USA and in Australia. Since it is simply a system which supports lip-reading, it can also be used with other spoken languages, and has been.

Fingerspelling is also frequently used to support spoken language. There is a one-handed system of fingerspelling and a two-handed. The two-handed is by far the most commonly used in the United Kingdom. By its means the 26 letters of the alphabet are represented by 26 hand positions. Using these hand combinations, the words of English can be spelled out. This is a somewhat laborious process and tends to slow down the process of communication when every letter of every word is signalled, although some users become remarkably proficient. For this reason some common words and certain proper nouns are indicated simply by the initial letter. Fingerspelling is frequently used in conjunction with spoken language to help clear up misunderstandings which may have occurred.

Another manual support system which is often used in combination with fingerspelling is *sign-supported English*. It is used principally with those who already have a good command of English, but who need more clues than they can get from spoken language alone. Signs taken from British Sign Language are used to supplement the spoken word, usually indicating the key words. The signs are of course used in the same order as English word order. In some situations the keyword signs are used without the words they represent being voiced, the 'listener' gaining the information from the sign, lip-reading and the context.

The manual support systems mentioned so far are mostly intended to be used in association with spoken language to provide additional clues. There are, however, support systems which are complete in themselves in that a full version of English is recoded into manual form. This is sometimes referred to as *manually coded English*. There are two principal types of manually coded English used in the United Kingdom, the *Paget Gorman Sign System* and *Signed English*. They are both intended to be used in combination with spoken language. The Paget Gorman Sign System was devised by Sir Richard Paget and was first brought to the fore as the New Sign Language in the early 1950s. It roots however were to be found in the 1930s when Prebendary Albert Smith put forward the view that young deaf children needed a new kind of sign language, one in which every sign would be a version of an English word and the signs would be made in the same order as the words of normal English speech, and with the same sentence construction. Sir Richard worked with his wife and others for more than eighteen years to construct such a systematic sign language. The signs which were devised were as far as possible pantomimic (i.e. they reflected in logical way the meaning of the word they represented). By 1950 or thereabouts approximately one thousand such signs had been invented and described, and the trial use of the New Sign Language which Sir Richard proposed was supported by Helen Keller no less! However, it wasn't until some considerable time later, after Sir Richard's death in 1955, that the system was further developed and refined by his widow and Dr Pierre Gorman. It was renamed 'A Systematic Sign Language' and a trial booklet which contained the fundamental principles and instructions for performing the signs for 1000 words was produced in 1966. This was replaced by a larger edition with 2000 words in 1969. Later the name of the system changed once again to its present name. It was introduced into several schools, together with a training programme and system of qualification for teachers. While it is still to be found in the United Kingdom, its use with deaf children has now largely disappeared.

The Paget Gorman Sign System did break new ground in that it provided a manually coded form of English for the first time in this country. By its means children were taught English through signs, although the signs were accompanied by speech. The theory was that, gradually, spoken English would in time take over and the signs would become redundant. One of the difficulties of such a system is being able to create enough distinct signs to cater for the rich vocabulary of the English language, but also the signs were not known by deaf adults. Consequently, those who failed to achieve mastery of spoken language were not able to communicate easily with hearing people or those deaf people who used British Sign Language. To overcome this difficulty Signed English was developed. This system adopted the principle established by Sir Richard Paget, that there should be an exact manual representation of spoken English, but instead of using invented signs, it used signs which were already an established part of British Sign Language. These signs are supplemented by some specially devised signs and 'markers' (to represent verb inflections, plurality, adjectival endings, etc.) and by two-handed fingerspelling, so that the grammatical features of English syntax can be properly incorporated. It is intended to be combined with speech, so that English is presented in an audio-visual form. Signed English is probably the most widely used form of the manual approaches in British schools.

TOTAL COMMUNICATION

While this is a term which is in wide use in this country and the United States, it is one for which it is difficult to find an acceptable definition. Indeed the British Association of Teachers of the Deaf in a policy statement on methods used in the education of deaf children in 1981 included definitions of all the major modes of communication to be found in our schools at that time. It said of total communication, 'A term in use for which there is no acceptable definition.' However, when it revised its policy document seven years later it was able to expand on this by stating:

> The term TOTAL COMMUNICATION may be applied to an approach to language acquisition and communication which uses combinations of oral, aural, written and manual components. The aural/oral components would be similar to those of the selected oral approach. Signed Supported English (British) and Signed English (British) are the most common manual components to be used in Total Communication.

In other words total communication is a mélange of a variety of different approaches and the 'mix' will vary from school to school, classroom to classroom and teacher to teacher. It may be used in different ways with different children in the same class and different teachers may use different combinations with the same child. The aim is to communicate with a child in any way that is possible—and anything goes. An American, Dr Roy Holcomb, is credited with giving the term 'total communication' to what he calls a philosophy rather than an approach or a method. David Denton, a fellow American working in the USA, who led the movement to promote it internationally has written that: 'Total Communication includes the full spectrum of language modes: child-devised gestures, the language of signs, speech, speechreading, fingerspelling, reading and writing.'

SIGN LANGUAGE

There are a number of sign languages used throughout the world, probably the most researched being American Sign Language and it is estimated that at least 75 per cent of deaf adults in America use it. Sign languages are languages in their own right, independent of other languages. They have their own vocabulary and grammatical structure and are used by separate communities. The signs themselves have at least four basic components: hand shape, orientation, location, and movement, and tend to represent broader concepts than the words of spoken language. There are physical constraints on the speed at which signs can be produced and perceived. Manual movements are much slower and less precise than the movements of the tongue and other speech organs, and it takes about twice as long to produce individual signs as it does to say words. So talking is faster than signing. Also visual perception is less effective than auditory perception when processing temporal (i.e. sequential) information. But sign language overcomes this problem by frequently producing what would be sequences in spoken language simultaneously. So some of the essential elements are produced together, rather than one after another. Also, the individual signs, being broader in concept, carry more meaning than individual words. The net result seems to be that the rate of expression of linguistic meaning is about the same as that of spoken language, so in practice it takes no longer to convey the same amount of information.

The sign language used by the deaf community in this country is *British Sign Language* which has been defined as a visual gestural language in terms of both its perception and projection. Gestures of the hands are used in combination with, and in relation to, body posture and facial expressions. Speech is not normally used to accompany the signing. British Sign Language owes much of its development to the education which was provided in residential special schools for the deaf, particularly during the last century. Most deaf pupils learnt it from their peers and their teachers rather than their parents, who in the great majority of cases were hearing, with no knowledge of sign language and little opportunity to learn it. The special schools using sign language frequently had their own unique signs, akin to dialect in spoken English, and these regional variations are still in evidence today. However, the detailed descriptions of the most commonly used signs, and the use of sign language on television in programmes for the deaf, will doubtless result in less diversity in due course. British Sign Language is thought to incorporate about 4,500 to 6,000 different signs. In comparison, the average adult English speaker uses a spoken vocabulary of about 15,000 words. Some of the signs are iconic, that is they convey a 'picture' of the object or idea which they symbolise, but many of the signs are purely arbitrary with no obvious relationship between the shape or movement of the sign and what it is portraying. The 'sign order' of British Sign Language is quite different from the word order of spoken English and while there have been attempts to use mimeographs of signs to record sign language on paper, sign language does not have a written form.

BI-LINGUALISM

Bi-lingualism is a more recent development in this country. There is some confusion about the precise meaning of the term 'bi-lingualism', some arguing that true bi-lingualism only occurs where the two languages are acquired simultaneously, this process starting before the age of two. Others make the distinction between primary language acquisition, secondary language acquisition and foreign language learning. However, in the current context it is the process whereby a child acquires British Sign Language as a first language and then either acquires, or is taught, English, with the emphasis on written English, as a second language. Sometimes when two languages are used together, at certain stages a mixture of both may occur in the language of the communicator. This type of mixture is sometimes referred to as 'pidgin'. Pidgins are not constructed systems but are the natural result of two languages being used together, usually by two hearing speakers who do not know each other's language. References to pidgin sign language and pidgin sign English are to be found in the literature, but these are not intended to be the outcome of bi-lingualism. The intended outcome of bi-lingualism is proficiency in two separate and distinct languages.

WHICH APPROACH FOR MY CHILD?

This is often the most difficult question the parents of deaf children have to answer. It is also the most difficult subject on which to obtain impartial advice, since most professionals involved in the education of hearing impaired children, or those who themselves are deaf, usually hold strong views. But at the end of the day it is parents who have to make the decision. The one piece of neutral advice which can be given is, 'Go to see the results of the various approaches used for yourselves.' However, before that can be a really useful course of action, parents need to know what to look for and even more important what the long-term goal of the education of deaf children should be.

What are we hoping to achieve when we educate our deaf children? The way this question is answered will determine the way in which we evaluate the various approaches which have been briefly outlined above. There can be two quite different long-term aims for deaf children. The first is that they should be educated so that they can become full, proud members of a deaf community, where they share with others the identity of being a deaf person. Although deaf people must of necessity spend time in contact with and within hearing society, many see themselves as deaf and as part of a separate minority culture. The second possible aim is that deaf children should be brought up to live in and see themselves as members of the hearing world, though not necessarily to the exclusion of the deaf community where some may wish to spend part of their leisure time. It is perhaps worth examining the approaches in the light of these two fundamentally different long-term goals for the education of deaf children, to try to determine which are likely to be the most successful.

Sign Language as a First Language

An essential requirement of belonging to a particular society is an ability to understand and to use the language that binds that society together, so for those parents who wish their offspring to grow up to belong to the deaf community first and foremost, this means a fluency in British Sign Language. Many of the parents for whom this is the fundamental aim, are themselves deaf and already members of the deaf community. They are likely to be fluent users of sign language and probably use this form of communication at home and in their social lives. Their children, be they hearing or deaf, will be exposed to this language from birth, and it will become their natural first language. Sign language will be acquired and will develop in much the same way that hearing children acquire spoken language from their hearing parents. Hearing children born into homes where sign language is used seem to have little difficulty in developing spoken English as they become progressively more exposed to it as they move out into the wider community through playgroups, nurseries and school. Deaf children from such homes will have more difficulty in this regard. Of course, for them the long-term goal of being able to take their place within the deaf community is well within reach, for these children will develop the language of that community. However, nobody would disagree that educational, vocational, leisure and social opportunities are considerably widened if these children can also develop a good knowledge of English. The big drawback of British Sign Language as an educational medium is that it does not have a written form, and it is difficult to imagine a 'book-free' system of education in the western world. So for these children a knowledge of English becomes essential. The big question is whether spoken or written English is the more important target. Usually, hearing children develop spoken language long before they learn to read and write, but is this the appropriate way round for deaf children who are already fluent sign-language users? Perhaps not. These children will have considerable difficulty in mastering spoken English, not least because it is unlikely that they will have used their residual hearing to the full in their early childhood. They would have been exposed to a silent language, and in such a world sound has less meaning. Their ability to be able to use effective amplification later on will depend to a great extent on the pattern and degree of their hearing loss. Those with a profound loss will have less chance than those with a severe loss. So perhaps learning written English first may be a better option, since it does not need the use of a defective and underdeveloped sense modality. There are numerous examples of hearing people who learn to read and write a foreign language with considerable ease, yet who never learn to speak it, and the situation of the sign language using child is not dissimilar. Certainly there have been historical suggestions that before oral education of deaf children became the norm, the written language of deaf people was better than it is today. Whether that was true for the majority of deaf people it is impossible to say. What we do know is that today the levels of literacy amongst the adult deaf population are considerably below those of hearing adults.

Bi-lingualism versus Total Communication

Of the approaches that we have considered, it is clear that, although it is as yet unproved in this country, *bi-lingualism* is the one most likely to benefit these children, with an emphasis on written English as the second language. For those children who have sufficient hearing to be able to develop spoken language by amplified listening, maybe placement in a wholly oral setting for their formal education would be appropriate, though it would be necessary to decide in each individual case whether structured oralism, the maternal reflective method or natural auralism would be the most appropriate. Certainly there are children who acquired British Sign Language from their parents as a first language, who have been successfully educated, and who have become reasonably fluent in spoken and written English in each of these three oral approaches. One thing that is clear, is that for this group of children total communication is unlikely to be of value. It is possible though, that Signed English, which is often used as the manual component of total communication, could be of benefit to some children as a way into written English.

However, deaf children of deaf parents are a tiny minority of the total number of children born with a hearing loss. Fewer than five per cent have two deaf parents (and not all of these will be sign language users), so the great majority of deaf children (over 90 per cent) will have hearing parents. A small number of these parents may decide that their deaf children will be able to live more secure and fulfilled lives as adults if they are able to live mainly with others who share their child's disability within the deaf community. But this situation is by no means as straightforward as it is for deaf children of deaf parents, because hearing parents use spoken language not sign language in the home. It is completely impractical to suggest that hearing parents could themselves learn to become fluent users of sign language sufficiently quickly for their child to be able to acquire sign language from them as a first language in the way most children acquire their mother tongue from their parents. Certainly it should be possible for parents who are well motivated to be able to learn sufficient signs for rudimentary communication in the early days to take place, but this will not be adequate for the development of language. Therefore, some artificial way of exposing the child for most of the day to British Sign Language has to be found. Several suggestions as to how this might be done have been made: having deaf people regularly in the home; having deaf 'linguistic mothers' who will be responsible for most of the early communication with the child; having the child fostered by deaf parents until the natural parents have been able to learn sign language; moving the child as soon as possible into a residential nursery where sign language is used. As we have already said many users of sign language learnt to use that language from their peers whilst at school, so placement in a special school where sign language is the language of the community would seem to be a good bet. In the past most special schools used a traditional oral approach as the method of teaching in the classroom and, in spite of this, sign language expertise was developed outside the classroom as children learnt from one another. How much greater the chance of an early fluency in sign language where this is the language used both inside and outside the classroom!

Total communication does not seem to be an appropriate approach if the goal is British Sign Language since, where it has any system to it, the 'system' leans more towards English than to Sign Language, and it is significant that in spite of the early acceptance of total communication by the deaf community many are now condemning it in favour of bilingualism. Harlan Lane, an American specialist in the psychology of language and linguistics, is a professor at Northeastern University in the USA who has spoken and written at length about the language and culture of deaf people. He dismisses total communication arguing that it destroys the grammar of sign language and effectively subordinates signing to speech. Wendy Daunt, Communication Consultant at the Royal School for the Deaf, Derby, examined the effect of total communication on children's achievements in school. She is reported to have found no improvement in their communication, education, British Sign Language, English, oral skills, social skills or reading age. She also considers that total communication, which she also refers to as 'total confusion' is unlikely to have a long-term future.[3] As a result of this work the school at Derby is abandoning its policy of total communication in favour of bi-lingualism. Bi-lingualism has also been adopted as the official policy of the Royal National Institute of the Deaf. While aiming for bi-lingualism the British Deaf Association, at the time of writing, still supports total communication as part of its official policy, but its director of sign language services, Liz Scott-Gibson, suggests that there may be a pragmatic reason for this since it may be a useful staging-post on the way to full bi-lingualism. So it would seem that the approach thought most likely to succeed with deaf children whose hearing parents want them to become members of the deaf community is that of bi-lingualism. Although experiments are taking place in one LEA, Leeds, to provide a bi-lingual approach within the framework of normal schools, it seems to us that this is much less likely to succeed than within the special school where the whole community can be British Sign Language users. In such an environment it should also be easier to have better control over the way the second language, English, is introduced and taught, particularly where written English is the main objective.

The great majority of hearing parents would prefer their offspring to be part of their own culture and society, and to be able to live comfortably in a hearing world. But if they are to be able to do this, they must become proficient in the understanding and use of spoken English. This must be their preferred mode of communication. Written English, while valuable, is not enough in itself. So when trying to decide which of the approaches to adopt when the long-term goal is living with hearing people, the first criterion must be how well does it lead to an understanding of spoken English and to an ability to talk intelligibly. And it is at the end of the period of compulsory schooling that this needs to be assessed. It should be obvious that this aim is easier to achieve where a child has more residual hearing. Nowadays, with early identification and the consistent use of the modern technology available to us to provide appropriate amplification, it should not be difficult to achieve where only a severe hearing loss (that is, an average loss in the better ear no greater than 95dB(HL) is present. The natural aural approach is the most obvious one to use for the majority of such children. For children with a profound loss it is more difficult.

Superficially, total communication seems an attractive option since, in theory at least, spoken information which is difficult to hear can be supplemented by visual clues in the form of signs. This manual support is likely to be Signed English or Sign Supported English. Unfortunately, results in this country have been disappointing if the goal is spoken and written English. Very few deaf children on total communication programmes in the UK develop a sufficient proficiency in spoken English for comfortable independent living in hearing society. The reasons why this seemingly attractive approach does not work well are no doubt complex. Clearly, if it is to be used from an early stage, parents will need to learn the manual signs which need to be used, almost certainly those of Signed English. This has a vocabulary of about 4,000 signs and 14 structural markers. While it is almost certainly easier to learn than British Sign Language, since it is after all only another form of English, it is still no easy task. Also, hearing parents typically use a spoken vocabulary which is three or four times that of Signed English. Whilst they may not use such an extensive vocabulary with young children, it is still likely that this will be considerably greater than that of Signed English. This means that, even where they have managed to learn all the signs, there will be frequent occasions when there is no corresponding sign for an English word or phrase which parents would normally use in a particular context. This presents a dilemma. Either they must use fingerspelling, which means slowing down the discourse and mastering another skill, or they need to simplify and paraphrase, thus reducing the richness and variety of the language being used. However, research findings (e.g. Bornstein[4]) suggest that parents of young deaf children frequently do not become proficient users of Signed English, and fathers in particular rarely get beyond the beginner stage. While this might be sufficient for the signalling of simple questions, demands or needs and for basic early communication, it hardly seems to be an adequate foundation for the acquisition of language, certainly not spoken language.

It also has been suggested that the brain has difficulty in processing both visual and acoustic information when presented simultaneously. One modality (usually vision) tends to dominate the other. But more important is probably the inability of the person 'speaking' to give a full and undistorted sequence of both sounds and manual signs simultaneously. As we have seen earlier, it takes much longer to form signs than it does to articulate words. Speech is about twice as fast. British Sign Language overcomes this difficulty because some of the information is presented simultaneously, but Signed English is simply a coding of English and therefore presents all information sequentially. This means that it takes at least twice as long to say anything! But we also know that the time relationships between the elements of speech are of very great importance. They carry a great deal of the underlying meaning. It is possible to render spoken language incomprehensible by deliberately altering its timing. Slowing speech down so that the signs can catch up with it destroys a great deal of this vital information. But it also appears that in order to try to keep up as fast a rate of speaking as possible, users of total communication unconsciously delete some of the signed component. Another problem is that of maintaining synchrony. This is extremely difficult to do. It also is the case that words and their corresponding signs do not always contain the same number of syllables. So words with one syllable in English may require two 'movement syllables' for the sign. We all know how disturbing it can be to watch a film of people talking where lip synchronisation has been lost. The auditory information is in conflict with the visual. In these circumstances people with normal hearing concentrate on the sound, trying to suppress the lip movements. In a total communication situation, if the signing falls out of synchrony, it not only conflicts with the auditory information, it also conflicts with the lip patterns. Which of these does the 'listener' tend to suppress? Probably audition and lip-reading, since the signing is more obvious and more dominant, particularly if you don't know the language very well anyway. So not only does this not help with the sounds of spoken language, it might actually hinder. It seems that the 'listener' receives two unsynchronised signals, each of which is incomplete and distorted. Rather than one supplementing the other, they probably interfere with each other.

So far we have concentrated on total communication as a possible means of developing spoken language in deaf children and what we have examined does not seem very encouraging. However, does this apply equally to written language? It is well known that many deaf children—and deaf adults, too—have difficulty with reading. Does total communication help in this respect? There is no evidence to suggest that it does. On the contrary the 1982-3 Gallaudet College survey of 55,000 deaf children reported a decline in their reading attainments compared to a similar survey twenty years earlier. It may of course be pure coincidence that in the intervening twenty years there was a major switch from oral-only programmes to total communication in the USA.

The arguments which apply to the use of Signed English as part of a total communication philosophy apply equally well to the Paget Gorman Sign System, and since it is difficult to find this system still in use with hearing impaired children in this country it is not necessary to discuss it further here.

Bi-lingualism is destined to become the approach which will replace total communication. However, even its advocates recognise that it may be unrealistic to expect deaf children to master spoken English following on from early years spent acquiring British Sign Language. Insufficient attention will have been paid to developing the use of residual hearing for linguistic purposes in those profoundly deaf children who acquire British Sign Language as their first language. The likelihood of their being able to develop proficiency in spoken language is remote. Researchers in the USA have stated recently:

> There is no evidence that a child can first become a competent signer and then learn to speak well. However, there is evidence that if you become a competent talker, you might later acquire signs if you wanted to be able to use both systems. Everybody we've ever studied who was competent with both modes, learned to speak first and sign later.

So it seems that if bi-lingualism is the aim for deaf children of hearing parents, then spoken language needs to be the first language.

Signs to Support English

Sign Supported English and fingerspelling cannot be considered as suitable approaches for developing spoken English in children, since their use presupposes an existing knowledge of English. Cued speech, however, has been widely used to support one or other of the oral approaches. It has now largely fallen out of use with deaf children in this country, where it is used in only one special school, and a handful of units, mainly in East Anglia. Teachers who have used this approach have found it more useful with severely deaf children than with the profoundly deaf. With the benefits of appropriate modern amplification, severely deaf children should not need this type of support; for profoundly deaf children it appears not to have worked, probably because the manual elements do not of themselves contain enough information, and its use disrupts the normal patterns of speech. While not having all the limitations of Signed English, the problem of cued speech is still that of speed and timing. While a small number of practitioners have been able to cue at commendable rates, for most adding cues to speech both slows it down and interferes with normal rhythm and intonation patterns.

Oral Approaches to Language Development

This leaves the oral approaches. *Traditional oralism* was in use for a long time and proved to be unsuccessful. In fact it was largely the failure of 'the oral method' as it was called, that gave rise to the renaissance of sign language in education in this country. The reasons for the failure of traditional oralism are now plain to see, since the way it sought to develop spoken language in children was, we now know, completely at variance with the way in which children acquire language. *Structured oralism* is a modern extension of traditional oralism, except that it places much greater emphasis on listening skills and these are considered to be at least as important as lip-reading skills. Much, but not all, of the language is structured and predetermined, but it is much more skilfully matched to the needs of children. Some of the children who have been educated through interventionist programmes of this type have been very successful. Their language is often more mechanical than natural, but it enables adequate communication with hearing people. For many it has provided an entrée into hearing society, and once there exposure to everyday language often has resulted in increased competence. Structured oralism is still to be found and a number of parents support it strongly.

The *maternal reflective method* and *natural auralism* are based on an entirely different philosophy to traditional and structured oralism. How successful are these approaches likely to be in producing young deaf adults able to use spoken English fluently? Both approaches are based upon spoken conversation as the main vehicle through which language is acquired by young children. The maternal reflective method is more interventionist than natural auralism. It also places much greater emphasis from an earlier age on the written word. Because it is based on group conversations, which are then written down and reflected upon, it is an approach which is more suited to a special school, or at least to a special class, of deaf children who are taught together as a group for much of the time. It has enjoyed considerable success, particularly with pupils who might be described as 'late-starting'. The

best example of its use in the UK is to be found at St John's
School, Boston Spa.

However, one of the latest approaches, natural auralism, has
provided the most spectacular successes—deaf young people
who use spoken English as their main means of
communication with a facility not hitherto achieved. While
not completely free from problems, independent living within
a talking community is clearly a realistic possibility. The main
problem with natural auralism is that, as with hearing
children, language is acquired primarily through the auditory
channel, even though this is the impaired modality. The
problems lay in providing and maintaining the high quality of
constant hearing aid amplification, which is essential if the
approach is to be successful, and preserving the naturalness of
the language of hearing parents whose child does not respond
in the way a hearing child does. The deafer the child, the
more difficult this is. As we have said earlier, there should be
little problem as far as severely deaf children are concerned,
but what has been so encouraging has been the number of
profoundly deaf children who have become fluent spoken-
language users. Parents, of course, need to play a major role.
It also takes a long time before the approach pays dividends
and parents need a great deal of faith and patience before
they can hear any results for themselves. While not a uni-
sensory approach, natural auralists believe that too great
attention to the visual presentation of information (e.g. by
signing) interferes with the development of the listening skills
which are necessary. There is evidence which supports this
view.

Another problem associated with natural auralism is the level
of skill required by the teacher. All approaches used with deaf
children are likely to be more successful where the teacher is
highly skilled. However, because natural auralism does not
appear to need anything out of the ordinary, such as fluency
in British Sign Language or Signed English, many teachers
feel that they can use a natural aural approach without the
need of special skills or study. This is far from the truth, and
many teachers who think they are using a natural aural

approach are not. Natural auralism is not, as yet, in widespread use with profoundly deaf children. It is used in four special schools, and a small number of LEAs, but it is our view that the results of the natural aural approach have been so encouraging, given the aim of independent living within a hearing world, that all parents should go to see the results of the approach before finally deciding which approach to adopt for their children. They can discover where they can see it in use by contacting the Natural Aural Group. The address is given in the Appendix.

Readers who may wish to delve into this fascinating subject to a deeper level than this brief overview of communication approaches used with deaf children can provide are recommended to read Lynas et al.[6] But for parents of deaf children there is no better means of making the right choice than by going to see the various methods in action and, above all, seeking the views of and communicating face to face with deaf school-leavers who have been educated by one or other of them.

Definitions

*Severe hearing impairment. A pure-tone hearing loss which in the better ear averages between 71dB(HL) and 95dB(HL) for the five octave frequencies 250Hz to 4kHz.

*Profound hearing impairment. A pure-tone hearing loss which in the better ear has an average of 96dB(HL) or greater for the five octave frequencies 250Hz to 4kHz.

For the purposes of calculating the average loss a 'no response' at any of the five frequencies is given the value of 130dB.

References

1 Van Uden, A. *A World of Language for Deaf Children,* 3rd ed., St Michielsgestel, 1977.
2 National Cued Speech Association of the USA, *Guidelines*

for the Definition of Cued Speach, reported in the Magazine section of the *Journal of the British Association of Teachers of the Deaf,* March 1990.

3   Report of 3rd annual National LASER Conference in *The British Deaf News,* January 1990, p. 7.

4   Bornstein, H. 'Signed English: A First Evaluation'. *Directions* 1, 3, (1980), pp. 21-2.

5   Westerhouse, J. 'Deaf education debate: signing vs the spoken word', *Medical Record,* 12:34, (1988).

6   Lynas, W., Huntington, A., and Tucker, I. G., *A Critical Examination of Different Approaches to Communication in the Education of Deaf Children,* Ewing Foundation, 1989. Available from Dr. W. Lynas, Dept. of Audiology, The University, Manchester M13 9PL.

4 The Range of Educational Options for Hearing Impaired Children

We should say at the outset that for a handicap so lacking in homogeneity as deafness, with its different types, different degrees of severity and differing additional problems, we believe that a broad range of educational provision should be made available for hearing impaired children. We should also say that as we outline the various forms of provision in this chapter you may well find that your Local Education Authority does not have available all the types we describe. In fact this would be very difficult if not impossible for individual authorities, particularly small ones, but we do believe that by sharing resources with others local authorities could and should make available much of the provision described below. If special educational needs differ then different resources are required to serve them. We have tried not to be too partial, i.e. not saying that one form of provision is always better than another, because it is not. It depends on the particular special educational needs of the child at that time.

Some parents will want to consider early nursery placement, perhaps even soon after diagnosis, taking the rational but unsophisticated view that the sooner the child has 'proper' classroom education the better. In our view what is required is as much time as possible interacting on a one-to-one basis with the main caregiver. It is important to remember that if diagnosis is late then the child may not have laid down the foundations of language which in normally hearing children would be set in the first year of life. This can only be done easily in a concentrated one-to-one interaction between parent and child and nowhere near so readily in the nursery or playgroup where adult attention is divided.

THE NURSERY SCHOOL.

Some of the claimed advantages of nursery education made by pioneers in that field would include the following:

1 Development of initiative, orderliness, sympathy.
2 Children become less bored and rebellious.
3 They are more independent of help from adults.
4 They develop a greater span of attention.
5 They develop more acceptable social behaviour.
6 They are more mature in their behaviour.
7 They have a better reaction to failure.
8 They become independent of adults earlier.
9 They develop more social contacts.
10 They become more outgoing and independent.

There has always been argument about how much children in nursery schools are there to be `taught' and to learn and how much the goals of nursery education are met through play and activity, Froebel being an early and staunch advocate of the latter. Other writers have argued that the nursery is a key bridge between the unrestrained life of play and the much more formal work of the classroom, and this late-19th-century view would probably hold sway in many quarters today.

 There is no doubt that the nursery education of handicapped children lagged substantially behind that of ordinary children—in the case of deafness not the least because the very late diagnosis took many children beyond the years of the nursery. By the end of the nineteenth century the United States had eight special schools for the pre-school education of the deaf, these being almost a hundred years behind those set up for ordinary children. In England in 1906 the average age of admission of the 43 schools for the deaf was greater than six years. J. Kerr Love, an advanced thinker of that time, considered that the loss of the years betweeen two and seven was an educational disaster, these years being the years in which speech and language are formed. Some recommendations he gave in 1910 would not go amiss in some uninformed parts of Britain in 1991:

1 Better medical diagnosis and follow-up.
2 Instruction for parents of young deaf children in their management and in the principles of speech and lip-reading.
3 Either:
  a The foundation of nursery schools to which the children would be taken daily, and to which the mothers would have free access, or
  b Peripatetic support to give some instruction to both parent and child.

Today there would be differences in emphasis—more on audition, qualifications, types of nursery, and so on—but Kerr Love's ideas seem remarkably fresh considering that they are eighty years old.

   In the late Twenties and Thirties a variety of types of nursery were set up with educationists seeing differing priorities, some to 'control and mould' and 'teach' in a didactic sense, and others to provide freedom and space, opportunities to gain experience of actual things, opportunities for social interaction, opportunities to learn skills in action rather than a concentration on abstract things. Lumsden, a very influential Inspector of Schools, stressed that experiences provide the base for the child's growing facility with language. In a sense Lumsden was telling us not to go overboard in these early stages trying to 'teach' the deaf child, yet many children were taken into very formal educational environments at three or even two years.

   The Forties saw debate on the purposes and values of nursery education for the deaf. There was a shift from test-oriented values—i.e. the view that if it is education then we should be able to test the improvement children make—to a more 'whole child' view, where the value of the nursery is seen not so much in the skills and knowledge that the children acquire but rather in their degree of 'educational readiness', their 'emotional stability' and their 'social adjustment'. Several writers saw the value of nursery education for the deaf as so important that they felt it should be available for every child.

Even in the Forties there was debate about the desirability of residential nursery placement and the danger that mother and child would achieve no satisfactory 'bond'. Certainly, later research suggested that prolonged separation from a caregiver before the age of three was potentially hazardous for the child's well-being.

It is fair to say that the pre-school area has been little researched over the years. It seems that researchers found it difficult to move from the early global 'it is a good thing' research, to more sensitive and specific investigation of aspects of nursery education. One study for the Warnock Committee investigating the education of the handicapped, however, did look at the benefits of and attitudes to nursery education for children with special needs. Since it was looking at the broad range of handicaps the number of hearing impaired children investigated was small. The study was carried out in the Central and Grampian regions of Scotland. The main findings, which revealed significant differences when comparisons were made with the interaction of normal childen, were summarised as follows: Handicapped Children—

1 were *more* likely to play *alone*.
2 were *less* likely to play with *other children*.
3 were *marginally* more likely to be *alone* with an adult.
4 spent a *similar* time in a group with an adult and children.
5 were *less* likely to engage in *imaginative* play.
6 were *more* likely to engage in *non-specific* activity or spend their time listening to or watching other activities.
7 were likely to communicate with adults and children for *similar* lengths of time.
8 were likely to communicate *less* with other children.
9 were likely to have *more one-way* than *two-way* speech patterns.

Amongst nursery staff, deafness was one of the handicaps which staff felt warranted special provision particularly if the deafness was severe. However, there was an admission that experience of the handicap was very limited—clearly a need for specialist professional support.

In another study carried out by staff from the Lancashire Service for Hearing Impaired Children the focus was on 11 hearing impaired children integrated into mainstream nurseries. The areas of communication, levels of maturity, use of hearing aids, school staff/parent relations and school staff/teacher-of-the-deaf relations were investigated. The children ranged from the partially to the profoundly deaf and the schools they attended ranged from 40- to 120-place nurseries. The results here seemed more promising and no serious problems were found. All the staff found that they were able to communicate with the children using speech, some natural gesture and by being willing to repeat instructions. All the hearing impaired children were found to be joining in and enjoying group activities especially those of a musical and action nature.

Two of the hearing impaired children were reported as more mature than the hearing children, while about a third were reported as less mature, in some cases, it was claimed, because of an 'over-protective family'. Three teachers said that the hearing children did not treat the hearing impaired children any differently but others suggested the hearing children's responses varied from treating them like everyone else, to treating them as scapegoats for problems, making allowances for them, treating them like babies, or ignoring them.

No significant problems were found with the use of aids although some of the nursery teachers complained of the 'wires getting caught up in the climbing frame' and others of the acoustic feedback from the aids. All the nursery staff gave favourable reports of the visits of specialist teachers of the deaf from the advisory service and said that most of the children had been well trained by their parents prior to entry in the areas of self help skills, toilet training and feeding behaviour.

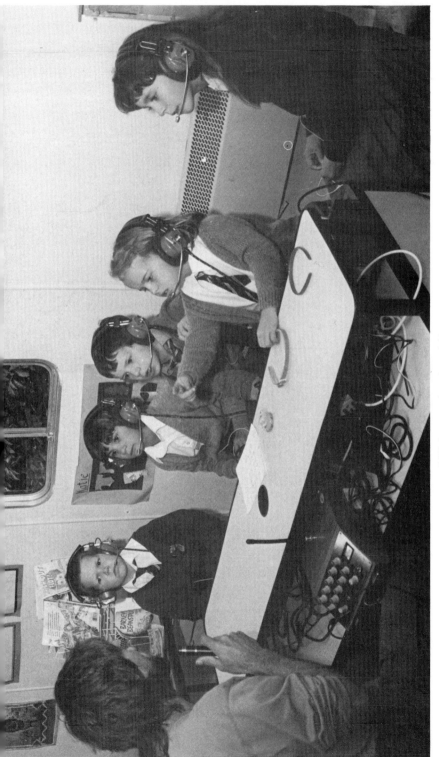

VIII A group hearing aid in use.

IX An auditory training unit.

It is of course difficult to draw firm conclusions from such research in view of the relatively small numbers of children involved in the studies but we hope to be able to point to some of the similarities in investigations to date.

There have been a few studies of the patterns of interaction of hearing impaired children placed in ordinary nurseries. One such study in Israel reported in 1985 that more profoundly hearing impaired children engaged in significantly less social integration than either severely hearing impaired children or normally hearing children. They also elicited fewer positive responses from hearing children, and engaged less in conversation than the severely hearing impaired children or the normally hearing children. British researchers, studying a nursery where eight hearing impaired children and 52 normally hearing children were on role, sub-selected, randomly, four of the hearing impaired and four of the normally hearing children to be observed by a time-sampling method. Observations were made of interactions with the teacher, interactions with normally hearing children, involvement with other hearing impaired children and of how much they engaged in 'watching' rather than active behaviour. The results were as follows:

1 The hearing impaired children were significantly more involved with the teacher than normally hearing children.
2 Normally hearing children approached and were approached by more normally hearing children than were the hearing impaired children. Also the approaches of the normally hearing children were more likely to be accepted.
3 The hearing impaired children were substantially more likely to be interacting with other hearing impaired children than were normally hearing children.
4 Watching behaviours of the two groups were similar.

Our observational experience suggests to us that the least successful nursery placements have been where there are several hearing impaired children in the same class. There was a period where schools for the deaf actually set up nurseries for their hearing impaired children and then drew in normally hearing youngsters to fill them up, or where a whole group of hearing impaired children were transported to the nursery school. In our view these were the least successful in achieving functional or real as opposed to merely locational integration. If the hearing impaired as a group have already established contact with hearing impaired peers it is nowhere near as likely that they will abandon these contacts in favour of breaking into the hearing circle.

One important study has looked beyond the interaction to the attitudes of the key adults on the scene—the parents, the teachers of the deaf and the teachers in the nursery. Ellen Bown[1] researching at Manchester University noted the Warnock Committee's statement regarding nurseries: 'First, the attitudes of the staff and the parents of all the children must be favourable.' It was felt likely that there would be overall differences in attitude and that knowing about these could aid the teacher of the deaf who is trying to anticipate potential areas of anxiety or feelings of inadequacy. She felt that there was always a danger of the teacher of the deaf becoming (because of experience) desensitised to the 'raw' reactions to hearing impairment—in this case, say, by the nursery staff. She felt that the specialist should do everything possible to understand the attitudes and feelings of the non-specialist.

In one section of the study, the main problems perceived by the teachers of the deaf related to communication and the use of hearing aids in noisy surroundings. Parents also mentioned communication problems but they stressed much more the the problem of the child adjusting to what was a new environment and of being *accepted*. Several expressed the fear that the nursery teacher would not have enough time for their child (a fear contrary to the evidence of most studies which show that the hearing impaired child seems to get more of the teacher's time than the normally hearing children) and would lack real understanding of the child's problems.

All three groups agreed that the major benefits of the nursery for the hearing impaired child would be the social and emotional advantages of the child having the companionship of children of the same age, the opportunity to develop normal play and behaviour patterns and the chance to become less dependent on mother.

As far as the child's social abilities are concerned teachers of the deaf mentioned a variety of problems including being isolated, possessive, demanding, withdrawn, self-centred, immature, aggressive and—*normal*. Nursery staff mainly reported the child as a withdrawn and insecure individual who tends to be aggressive because of the frustration caused by his handicap. Parents were in close agreement, mentioning shyness, isolation and frustration.

On language development nursery staff were positive that benefits would accrue, while the teachers and parents were fairly equally divided into three groups, those who:

1 felt the nursery would make a valuable contribution to natural language;
2 felt that nursery might help but that interaction with the parent and teacher were more important; and those who
3 felt that the nursery would not make any difference at all to language development.

Bown's study was interesting in that it brought out differences in attitudes to normal nursery placement, teachers of the deaf being most positively in favour, followed closely by the nursery teachers with the parents of the hearing impaired children themselves being more variable in their attitudes and having the most reservations about normal nursery placement.

Attitudes towards the following aspects were investigated:

1 Special needs.
2 Benefits from normal nursery/local treatment.
3 Handling problems.

4 Concern for how the deaf child would fit into the nursery.

5 Being away from home.

For each of the above factors there were differences between parents and teachers of the deaf, with teachers of the deaf being more positive. Also, with the group of parents there was much more variation in attitude than there was in either of the two teacher-groups. Briefly, regarding the above aspects the following attitudes were shown:

* Special needs: nursery teachers and teachers of the deaf were similar in attitude and felt competent to handle the situation, but parents had varying views and more reservations.
* Benefits: the parents showed a great deal more uncertainty.
* Problems: for the only time the nursery staff were more positive than the teachers of the deaf.
* Concern and absence from home: perhaps predictably parents were less positive and a great deal more "uncertain", working as they were with little knowledge of other deaf children who had been successfully integrated into an ordinary nursery.

Bown's study highlights for us the need for those who support the parents of young hearing impaired children to carry parents with them when they give advice. We have to be convincing in our arguments and as far as possible correct in our judgements. In the study described it seems that the parents were not always convinced of the efficacy of proposals made by their advisers. It was also made clear in the study that while it was thought that the nursery specialist was the one with the specialist expertise in handling very young children, there was a great need for there to be readily available specialist support for the placement by teachers of the deaf. We would envisage the support including the following:

1 The advisory teacher should provide the specialist support for the child's amplification systems, undertaking regular checks, both simple and electro-acoustic (using a hearing aid test box), frequently and regularly.
2 The great majority of sensori-neurally hearing impaired children should be fitted with FM (radio transmission) systems in order to offset as much as possible the very adverse noise conditions found in most nurseries.
3 The teacher of the deaf should ensure that the hearing impaired children are fitting into the educational environment by, if necessary, carrying out observational studies of the interaction within the classroom.
4 The teacher of the deaf should provide in-service training so that the nursery staff are aware of what deafness means to the child, how to handle hearing aids, put earmoulds in, not talk when looking away from the child, etc.
5 The teacher of the deaf should continue to support the family of the hearing impaired child at home, bearing in mind that he will spend more time there than in the nursery.

Of course it is advantageous for the hearing impaired child to be exposed to normally hearing children of the same age, size and with similar interests and talking to him at his level, but it is possible to overestimate the importance to language development of a nursery placement. It was interesting in the Bown study that both professionals and parents emphasised social and emotional factors above language development as the value of the nursery. We believe that language is learned at the mother's knee and that it is in the home that much time can be spent providing opportunities for meaningful linguistic exchanges.

We believe that the child who is perhaps not diagnosed until a year or eighteen months (an unpleasant fact but a frequent one still in this country) should be delayed in entering a nursery in order to give time to get used to amplification and to engage in the activities in the home which lay down the ground rules for language development. *The child should go to the nursery with an already developing language system, not in the hope of starting one off.* Great care should be taken in the placement and note should taken of how much of the time at the nursery is spent by adults talking with children and how much those adults spend their time in paperwork, talking to other adults, putting out and taking away equipment and in supervising as opposed to talking to children (see Plates XVIa and b).

In the late Sixties professional organisations concerned with hearing impaired children were still campaigning for special nurseries for such children. But by the mid-Seventies new nurseries which had been built were difficult to fill and many of the existing ones had closed. Today very few special nursery classes for the deaf remain. Why this dramatic change? It seems to have been caused by two principal factors, a recognition of the value of young hearing impaired children mixing with their hearing counterparts and a reaction to sending very young children away from home to residential schools. Although, as we have noted above, not without drawbacks, the activities of a vibrant ordinary nursery environment were seen to benefit hearing impaired children socially and linguistically. Children so placed compared favourably with those in special nursery classes, so why send them away from home with the possibility of weakening the emotional attachment to the family and the risk of adverse reaction?

PREPARATION FOR SCHOOL

Whether the child is starting school for the first time, changing schools or moving into a boarding situation for the first time there are many things that will help to prepare for the new situations to be faced as they take their place alongside the other children.

If it is the child's first school much time will be spent playing, but it should not be assumed that the time is being wasted, since play is children's work and it is through play that they learn. Common activities might be building with bricks of different sizes; play with water and sand; classifying and sorting objects; weighing and sorting beads and nuts etc; and playing at shops. All these things help children to learn important relationships relevant to their understanding of mathematics. In a similar way imaginative and creative play is important in helping them to develop natural language and communicative skills. All the activities mentioned above help to further development of language and demand that children co-operate with each other.

Play

Singing and saying rhymes and listening to stories are important in encouraging verbal skills, and these activities also act as transmitters of our culture. In doing these things the child really feels part of a group, probably for the first time, and great delight is taken in interacting with classmates. Children do these and many more things in the classroom, so it is obviously useful if they can already play constructively both on their own and with small groups of other children. This cannot be achieved overnight so it is best if parents themselves play a lot with the children and gradually introduce them to others by taking them to play with neighbours' children as well as inviting children back to their own home.

Play is a sufficiently important topic to be dealt with in a book of its own but it is worth mentioning that play has its uses in developing many of the skills and attitudes which are so important when a child goes to school.

Separation

Separation has to be dealt with on many levels including the separation when the child goes away to a residential special school. This is never easy—even the first day at the local nursery can bring tears to both child and parent, but it is helpful if the child has, during the pre-school period, been gradually prepared for separation. He should be encouraged to spend time with friends and relatives, thus getting the idea that separation happens but that you always return.

Sharing and Turn-taking

Activities which encourage the child to share and take turns are very good preparation for school. Children should be taught to share sweets and to use toys communally, as well as to play games such as lotto, snakes and ladders, dominoes and so on where a group of people play and take turns. It is important that children are not always allowed to win, since learning to lose gracefully is important, but a parent may be forgiven for manipulating enough success to keep the child interested and motivated.

Learning Good Manners

The child should be encouraged to say 'please' and 'thank you' and not to snatch things when handed them. A useful anti-snatching ploy is to make the young child sit when receiving things. This is obviously very useful with things such as food and drink, but it can be extended to other things too, since it is much more difficult to snatch when sitting. However parents try to tackle this problem it is most important that they are consistent. If it is naughty to snatch then it is naughty every time and snatched items should be removed. Then, of course, when the child takes things nicely he or she is rewarded with a smile and 'that's a good boy or girl'.

Storytelling

Storytelling has always occupied a key position in the school day and it is very valuable if children new to school are not also new to books, both from the point of view of handling them with care and from knowing some of our favourite traditional stories. At the start parents can use such stories as 'The Three Little Pigs' which is very high on visual content and where the child can take part in acting-out the 'huffing and puffing'. Another very good story is the 'Three Billy Goats Gruff', but the list is endless and parents should have no difficulty in finding wonderful stories to tell their children in the same way as the teacher at school will tell them. It is good to tell the stories in your own words and use the pictures in the book to illustrate, and it is vital that they are told with lively expression. As children become familiar with the stories they can be encouraged to take part in acting them out and eventually they will want to tell the story themselves, so it is helpful if there is someone around who is ready to listen! It is easy in our desire to stimulate hearing impaired children with natural language to forget that they also want to communicate with us. Watch for the child's attempts—listening is most important.

Many teachers in ordinary schools say that many young children do not know how to sit quietly and listen either to stories or to instructions, and some blame the almost continuous noise of music and television. With hearing impaired children we think it is even more important to have quiet times through the day and to use television constructively so that parents and children can all take part in the interesting range of programmes available.

Developing Reading and Writing Skills

At this point we are not suggesting that parents teach their child to read and write, but it is true to say that many of the games that well-motivated parents play with the young child will also be encouraging visual development and fine control of fingers. Thus painting and crayoning are helpful for later writing skills as is writing the child's name on his or her pictures in large lower case letters, a good stimulus for visual recognition.

It is our view that the early emphasis should be on encouraging listening and talking skills. As far as listening activities are concerned the following are very useful:

1 Copying clapped patterns, as in some nursery rhymes.
2 Making a noise with an object the child cannot see, and asking him or her to identify it.
3 Making pictures or stories in sound: some of these can be obtained on tapes, ranging from the simplest noise of a fire engine to quite complicated sound stories. Sound stories also help the child to think in sequence.

4 Playing with puppets, mime and drama encourages the child
  to be more relaxed and outgoing.

Allied to the above there is always the need to give children
plenty of opportunity to tell you things. They can be
encouraged to tell their own stories and to show an interest in
nature, science and any other topic likely to stimulate
conversation.

Activities which have the benefit of extending vocabulary are
endless but parents and teachers should remember that nouns
are easy and so should not have too much emphasis. Words
should be used in as many contexts as possible so that the
child comes to appreciate that the same word can be used in
many ways.

Children should be encouraged to look carefully and in
detail at pictures and objects. They should be asked questions
which require this careful observation. The idea of sequence,
which is important in encouraging children to read from left
to right for instance, can be further stressed by use of picture
stories (some comic strips are good for this). Children should
be encouraged to think: they should not be just asked what *is*,
but what *is not*, what *is missing* and what *is different?* Encourage
children to match pictures. Parents and teachers can build up
a collection of their own with lots of duplicates so that they
can say, 'Find me another cat!', 'Is there another tree?' and so
on. Picture lotto, picture dominoes, snap, happy families, lost
and found, also encourage this skill. These kinds of games can
be linked with development of one-to-one correspondence in
mathematics, where one item, say a picture of one saucer, is
matched to a picture of one cup.

As far as the actual reading of words and sentences is
concerned, it may be useful if we outline our views and make
a few suggestions. Teachers talk of 'reading readiness', and if
this concept is to have any meaning then we would take it to
be the point where the child has matured sufficiently, or has
enough previous learning, to enable him to proceed easily
with learning the skills of reading. There is certainly plenty of
evidence to suggest that activities such as we have described,

which improve children's visual and auditory discrimination, help them towards readiness to read. In the early years we often limit the child's language experience to the experience of spoken words, but there is good evidence that the same early period should be used for the mastery of visual language symbols.

In saying this we are not contradicting our view that parents should not be involved in early formal instruction. We do not believe that parents should be using formal reading schemes—not because we do not believe that only the teacher can do this, but because this is not where reading should start. Reading should start from the child himself and his or her own experiences, and not from second-hand experiences in printed books. In other words in the period before entry to school the best approach is to devise an environment in which children learn to read in the same way as they 'learn' to talk, *naturally*.

A good place to start is with the child's own name. A large book can be made with a picture of the child on the cover. The parent can write (in a balloon coming from the child's mouth) 'I am Peter' (or 'I am Jane'). The child can be asked to read it with the parent. Similar writing can be associated with other pictures of mummy or daddy or other members of the family. Work can done on 'I can', 'I have', and soon the child can gradually be encouraged to do his or her own drawings, and to ask for words. Whatever is written for children should be in the lower case, as follows:

a b c d e f g h i j k l m n o p q r s t u v w x y z

This is very important because it is what the teacher will use in school, and what the child will see in any printed book. It is also helpful if in the early stages parents write large clear letters.

Alongside the above parents might also encourage children to read labels, such as 'television', 'video', 'chair' and so on, by sticking labels on these items and then getting the child to match further labels to them, and to read the words. They can also be encouraged to attempt to read the many labels in everyday life and make a collection: 'cornflakes', 'honey', 'butter', 'milk', 'stop', 'wait', 'car park', 'bus stop' and so on.

As children's interest develops they may be encouraged to produce their own scrapbooks of *the living room, the kitchen, the garage, the zoo, the park, the seaside,* using pictures from old magazines, catalogues, and postcards. Parents write in the appropriate words and the books become the first reading books for the child. Parents can even make flash cards which the child can use to match to words in the books. This works best if both the scrapbooks and the flash cards are large with large print. This is an approach that both writers have used with their own children and with hearing impaired children and it gives an opportunity to develop quite a large reading vocabulary without any resort to a reading scheme. It pays always to be guided by the child, since if you push too hard it will seem to be a chore and the child will react adversely, but if it is done sensitively the child will come for more and more words and be delighted to demonstrate the growing skill at reading them.

Children can be encouraged in writing-related skills, copying wavy lines and a variety of shapes. If they attempt to draw over the 'writing patterns' then they should be encouraged and complimented, but if not they should be left to do their own drawings and paintings. It is very helpful to have large sheets of paper, fat crayons and thick paint brushes.

The tactics described above are those which will encourage *word recognition,* but this stage in reading is the easiest one, and many children will appear to read before they are actually able to do so in the true sense. The task of parents and later teachers is to ensure that the reading of words goes hand-in-hand with the child's understanding of those words. Parents should certainly forget any thoughts they may have that children are only learning reading when they are being formally instructed from a reading scheme. They, like teachers, should be encouraging children to see the words all around them.

INTEGRATION IN THE MAINSTREAM

The Peripatetic Service for Hearing Impaired Children

In Britain this is also called the 'advisory' teaching service, or 'visiting' teacher service and covers support for the families of pre-school hearing impaired children and those placed in mainstream schools without a special resource unit. In the United States such teachers are called 'itinerant' teachers.

In some cases a whole service including peripatetic service, partially hearing or special resource units and even a special school are united under a single head of service. *We are very much of the opinion that unified support for hearing impaired children is vital.* If well run it is better geared to service delivery according to need and is much more likely to allow flexibility in the type of provision offered to the child. From a staff point of view it can more easily offer career structure and a sense of being part of a team. Procedures can be laid down for children to have regular reviews, audiological support throughout the whole audiological service and there being a 'service' for hearing impaired children means that its head can fight in the corridors of power for a proper share of scarce resources along with other special needs interests.

There is difficulty in ascribing a single name mainly because of the wide variety of roles such teachers fulfil, from counselling and guiding parents of very young children; advising teachers of ordinary children who have a hearing impaired child in their class; to visiting the hearing impaired child in the ordinary school to carry out remedial micro-teaching. For some there are other tasks as well, such as participating in multi-disciplinary diagnostic teams; providing short courses for all kinds of interested and involved personnel; supporting students in further education and higher education; and supporting hearing impaired children in other types of schools, e.g. schools for children with physical and mental disorders.

In view of the nature of this book we shall focus on how

they support ordinary teachers and help children who are placed in mainstream classes.

MANAGING AND TROUBLESHOOTING CHILDREN'S HEARING AIDS
This is a key function of the peripatetic teacher and involves checks that they must do and checks that they must train the mainstream classroom teacher to do. Most of the latter checks are very simple to carry out and it is better if they are carried out daily and recorded on an appropriate sheet. (See Chapter 2 which deals with this issue in detail.)

In-service Training of Mainstream Teachers

Mainstream teachers need to be aware of the types of amplification system used by deaf children and the ways in which certain environmental conditions can limit their effectiveness. This we cover in detail in Chapters 2 and 7. The way teachers control children in their classroom is of paramount importance for a child with a hearing loss. Clearly the classroom where children stop and listen carefully when instructions are being given are more 'environment friendly' than classrooms where teacher instructions compete with already existing child noise. They also need training in the management of hearing aids and on-going access to the specialist teacher of the deaf for support in their use in the classroom. Teachers in the mainstream should also have a basic understanding of the anatomy and physiology of the ear and hearing as described in Chapter 1. They will also require information on the likely effects on learning of a hearing loss. Teachers in the primary school have few, if any, free periods and it may be difficult for a school to provide cover for the training to take place. But these are difficulties which need to be overcome, for if the training does not take place then the child's special educational needs will not be met.

Ordinary teachers will need to know that how they make their comparisons between hearing and hearing impaired pupils is very important. For example, direct comparison of a child's educational achievements with those of hearing children is valuable but is NOT the key issue. A more relevant comparison is that between the child's educational, social and emotional progress with that of other hearing impaired children who have similar hearing losses and who are placed outside the mainstream. The ordinary class teacher may well need the help of the specialist teacher to be able to make this comparison. It would be quite easy for the mainstream teacher to feel that the hearing impaired child is failing when in fact he is far outstripping his peers in alternative placements. The key to the ordinary classroom teacher being well informed is a very knowledgeable specialist teacher of the deaf.

INTERACTION IN THE CLASSROOM AND LIP-READING

In terms of interaction within the classroom we believe that teachers should be aiming as closely as possible for a normal situation but there is no doubt that on questions such as lip-reading there are guidelines that can help. Much is claimed for lip-reading but it is at best imprecise and only an aid to what the child can hear through hearing aids. Two-thirds of the sounds that make up the English language are not easily seen or else are visually ambiguous. Many are greatly dependent on voicing and nasality for them to be understood. Since these features are not directly visible various groups of sounds such as 'p', 'b', 'm'; 't', 'd', 'n'; and 's', 'z' are liable to frequent confusion. Some other consonants, e.g. 'k', 'g', 'y', are produced far back in the mouth and are virtually invisible. Another feature of speech which adds to the difficulty of lip-reading is that it is very rapid and impermanent. There is a distinct possibility that lip-reading is one of the many skills which heavily rely on innate capacity and is not very amenable to training. It is our view that lip-reading will support the child as he builds his system of speech and language but that his requirement of it and dependence on it will be governed to a large extent by his early experiences. We believe that early and appropriate fitting of high-powered amplification has meant that such children are much less reliant on visual cues for communication and develop their language auditorily—hence some children at the Mary Hare Grammar School can, with appropriate amplification, communicate perfectly well on the telephone in spite of average hearing losses in excess of 100dB(HL). Children do take cues from the face and gesture to aid their residual hearing and there is evidence that auditory/visual reception is superior to that of audition and vision separately, but each child must personally determine the amount of visual information required. How much, this will be depends on many factors, including the degree of deafness, the age hearing aids were fitted and their appropriateness, and the environment in which the child is trying to listen.

It is helpful if teachers remember:

1 Lip-reading is easier in good light levels.
2 Lip-reading is difficult if the subject is in silhouette against a very bright window.
3 Lip-reading is very difficult if the teacher is a 'pacer i.e. paces up and down the classroom while talking to the children.
4 Lip-reading is impossible if the teacher is facing the blackboard while speaking!
5 Lip-reading is easier if the teacher speaks naturally with clear enunciation and at a natural pace. Exaggerated speaking and movement of lips is not at all helpful, neither is whispering, nor shouting, since they destroy the natural rhythm and intonation of speech.
6 As a good backup to audition and lip-reading it can be very helpful if the teacher is able to jot down major ideas on an overhead projector.
7 It is important that the teacher should frequently check on what the deaf child is getting from the discussion. Teachers must not simply assume because the child nods his head in response to a question such as 'Do you understand?' that he actually is following the discussion. The teacher must check by requiring an answer containing specific information.

8   The teacher can help the child with a hearing loss by 'reflecting back' answers given by other class members since the teacher using the radio transmitter may be the only person in the classroom who is well heard by the child.

9   The teacher should be aware that for the child with a hearing loss concentration on listening and watching is very tiring and, wherever possible, difficult-to-follow lessons should be held earlier in the day and lessons which require deep concentration should be interspersed with lessons where the children themselves are active. This is of course true for all children but much more so for the hearing impaired child.

10 The child should wear his personal hearing aids at all times except in the swimming pool. In the mainstream classroom there may be additional occasions where the radio reception system is too bulky to be worn, e.g. in the gymnasium.

THE TEACHER'S ATTITUDE TO SPEECH AND LANGUAGE

We are absolutely convinced that mainstream teachers have no role to play in formal speech correction work, since they have no training for this. Within the mainstream environment the aim must be to stimulate hearing impaired children with natural language. Unskilled speech intervention with hearing impaired youngsters can do untold damage. We also know that in some authorities mainstreamed children are being supported by sign interpreters. We are not clear how this can be described as 'integration' when the child must pay most attention to a 'specialist' signing the content of the lesson, and not to following the mainstream teacher. It is then difficult for the child to take part in pupil-to-pupil interaction and really become part of the class. The question must be asked whether children who require the use of sign language would not be better served by being placed in a special school where sign language is the medium of communication and where all lessons are delivered in that medium by specialists.

Any formal speech work for a child placed in the mainstream would, if required, be carried out by the teacher of the deaf or a speech therapist, but mainstream teachers in order to liaise effectively with advisory teachers should be aware of the more common speech faults they are likely to come across. Articulation may be defective in one or more of the following areas:

1 Omissions—where a sound is left completely out of a word, e.g. 'ga–' for 'gas' or 'bu–' for 'bus'.
2 Substitutions—where one sound is used in place of another, e.g. 'wed' for 'red' or 'tat' for 'cat'.
3 Distortions—where an approximation of the sound is used, e.g. 'bwake' for 'brake' or 'mash' for 'match'.

Among the more frequent errors in the speech of hearing-impaired children are the omissions of high-frequency sounds, which they find most difficult to hear because their hearing loss is most severe in those regions and because those sounds are among the least intense in speech e.g. 's', 'p', 't', 'f'. What is quite amazing is how many manage to learn to produce these sounds by a mixture of hearing and visual clues or with a little help from a specialist teacher or speech therapist.

Developing any language depends on exposure to a fluent and tuned version of that language within everyday interactions. In more than 90 per cent of cases both parents of the hearing impaired child are normally hearing, so sign language will not be used in the home. In all mainstream schools the medium of instruction is English, so sign language is not the language of the school. No sensible or realistic person believes that normally hearing children are going to learn sign language to a proficient level simply in order to communicate with deaf signing children in a mainstream school, so logic dictates that mainstream children should be talking children.

We are not saying 'no sign language for any child', we are saying that the population of deaf people is a very heterogeneous one and that the great majority are capable of speaking and spend their everyday lives surrounded by spoken language. For those who, usually because of a combination of factors, are not able to use spoken language, placement in a special school, where specialist teachers fluent in sign language can teach them, is essential if a child's education is to proceed satisfactorily.

It is clear that the service for hearing impaired children needs to use speech and language evaluation techniques both to help in deciding on the level of integration afforded to each child and also to monitor progress in that provision. This might well include a sample of free speech videoed or taped along with the use of tests such as the GAEL test (Grammatical Analysis of Elicited Language), the EPVT (English Picture Vocabulary Test), the TROG (Test for the Reception of Grammar) and the EAT (Edinburgh Articulation Test). As with most tests there are problems (for example, the EPVT is not a good test of progress) but taken together very useful information can be gleaned about the child.

OTHER FORMAL TESTING PROCEDURES
In order for services for hearing impaired children to make the decisions about whether they will integrate the child, and if so to what level, we feel that they need information on all of the following:

1 Intellectual ability.
2 Hearing loss.
3 Handicaps additional to the hearing impairment.
4 Language development (including syntax, grammar and vocabulary).
5 Speech intelligibility.
6 Hearing-aid use (regularity, care, willingness to wear a radio aid, speech tests in noise, aided threshold tests).
7 Mathematical ability.
8 Reading ability.

The Partially Hearing Unit

A partially hearing unit (PHU) or unit for hearing impaired children is to be found in most local education authority areas, but this title is now quite misleading since many units contain children with severe or profound hearing losses. The first four such units were opened in London in 1947. They were the result of progress made in early diagnosis and use of amplification with moderately deaf children. They were set up in primary schools, it being the aim that by the time the children reached secondary age they would have developed sufficiently well to be able to attend ordinary schools. The idea was that if the children did not reach the required standards by that time they would be transferred to special schools for the partially hearing.

The original Department of Education and Science definition of such a 'unit' was a 'group of partially hearing children which is being educated in any one school, which also has children of normal hearing, and is under the care of one or more teachers of the deaf appointed for the purpose. A unit may consist of one class, several classes or a number of individual pupils distributed amongst the ordinary classes, who return to the special teacher for tutorial periods.' (See Plate XVII.)

In the early days the statutory maximum number of children in the unit was ten. Now there is no statutory figure but ten rapidly came to be seen as too many when consideration was given to the often complex and difficult teaching circumstances of the unit. One very common problem was that with deafness being such a rare handicap the unit would have a very wide age-spread in its children, making effective teaching very difficult. Where integration for part of the time into the mainstream classes was planned it was noted that the school could be too small to absorb the children from the unit. Most people would agree that the hearing impaired child demands additional individual attention and that it is possible to 'over-weight' a class with such children.

However, in our view a prime goal of the unit must be to integrate the children into ordinary classes as far as possible, while having the unit and its specialist teacher on hand for specialist support. The opportunity is thus provided to support the child in the mainstream class or withdraw him or her to the unit for specialist teaching. There has always been the question, 'What is the child missing in the mainstream while he is being taught in the unit?' And there has been evidence that in some areas they have been missing a great deal, some subjects not appearing on their timetable at all. Religious Education, Music and French are the most frequently omitted subjects but Powers[2] has found that even Technology, History and Geography are omitted for some pupils in some units. The National Curriculum now demands a broad balanced curriculum for every child and teachers will have to think very carefully before withdrawing a child, because they will need to ensure that the child still has access to all the subjects on the curriculum.

NCC wishes to reaffirm this principle of active participation by the complete range of pupils with Special Educational Needs (including those with profound and multiple learning difficulties), whether they are in special, primary, middle or secondary schools, with or without statements.

(National Curriculum Council Circular 5, para. 3).

Powers also noted that only 48 per cent of hearing impaired pupils were following six or more GCSEs in partially hearing units and 25 per cent were following three or less and 8 per cent none at all. Of especial interest in this study is the high level of individual teaching carried on in units. In 1967 a DES survey reported 67 out of 74 units 'functioned as classes' while Powers found that only seven out of 122 units were taught as classes. Thus support is provided in the ordinary class as well as individually in the unit. A slightly worrying feature of the study was that many heads of unit felt that it was more problematic to organise in-class support than withdrawn support; also that many pupils felt happier about going to the unit than about unit staff going in to lessons with them. Many heads of unit thought that class teachers did not welcome in-class support. More worrying still was that in many schools unit staff were being used to cover mainstream class teachers. One certainly wonders whether unit teachers have sufficient training to help mainstream teachers and if not whether an 'umbrella' service for hearing impaired children in the particular district is adequately equipped to provide service. Another worrying feature is the fact that 38 per cent of units in the Powers study were staffed by only one teacher, making those units very vulnerable to staff absence. Seven per cent had no teacher of the deaf in them.

Returning to the curriculum within units, it will be possible for hearing impaired children to be taught outside the set stages of the National Curriculum for their age level and the more severely handicapped will certainly need this if their educational needs are to be met. However, far more than ever before this will need to be justified in the child's statement of special educational need. We believe rightly so.

In some schools there may be opposition from ordinary class teachers to having a handicapped child in an already overcrowded class. Class teachers, with the moves towards greater integration, are now having increased demands placed on them. The wife of one of the present authors has a class of more than thirty infant children one of whom is severely hearing impaired, another is severely behaviourally disturbed and another is markedly slow learning. It is thus vital that unit teachers are not seen by the rest of the school as merely having a 'soft option' in working with a very small number of children, but as hardworking members of the whole school. This raises the question of whether they should be 'attached' (solely responsible to the head of the mainstream school) or 'unattached' (where they are responsible to the head of the school on a day-to-day basis but have a main responsibility to the head of service for hearing impaired children).

We believe that they should, wherever possible, be attached to a service for hearing impaired children because of the very real dangers of professional isolation. Isolated teachers can swiftly lose track of what is possible with hearing impaired children and this leads to outdated ideas and low expectations for their children. They also require the expert support of the educational audiologist and appropriate technical support to help them maintain their amplification equipment at peak efficiency.

The main problem for the partially hearing unit is that it can become much like a mini special school, being effectively isolated from the rest of the school and yet not having the advantages of a special school, i.e. a larger and mutually supporting staff, good audiological backup and often good technical support. The units in the Leicestershire service have been reduced in number in favour of individual integration in local schools, but those which remain are supported by a county-wide service including several audiologists and a first-rate technical team. In the Leicestershire units the children spend a substantial portion of their time in ordinary classes. This, like many services, has seen big changes in its unit clientele, the children now so placed being more severely hearing impaired than a few years ago. There is movement into the unit system for children in need of increased support and out again into the mainstream when that additional support is no longer required.

Earlier diagnosis and good pre-school work have led to the above changes and it is now not uncommon in Leicestershire and other good services to see children with very severe hearing losses being placed directly into the mainstream. A key advantage of mainstreaming is that the child attends a school close to home with children who are neighbourhood contacts and friends. This, in our view, is a key problem of the static unit which has specially developed facilities as a special class within an ordinary school (a room or rooms of quiet within a noisy mainstream school!). The unit is often located in a particular school where there has happened to be a spare room capable of conversion, or where the head was known to be supportive of the principles of integrating handicapped children. Unfortunately, this classroom is often not in the school closest to where the hearing-impaired child lives so one of the main objectives, social advantage, can be missed. Unit children are frequently taxied to a distant school and have little or no opportunity for out-of-school contact with fellow pupils. The children also have more difficulty in participating in extra-curricular activities.

The Manchester Education Authority have been trying an idea they call the 'resource base' where the child is identified as a pre-schooler and his neighbourhood school is resourced with some facilities which, though not of the high standard of a fixed partially hearing unit, do enable the child to be placed in a local school with specialist teacher support. We understand that not all necessary schools can be so resourced, so some children still have to travel to a resource base for their education. This more flexible unit would then be disbanded once the children had moved through to the next stage of education. The aims of flexibility are commendable, providing appropriate children are placed in what must be a lightweight form of provision, lacking as it is in careful acoustic treatment and specialised amplification fitting.

THE SPECIAL SCHOOL

When people come to consider a special school as opposed to mainstream or unit placements, then there are various options available according to the special needs of the child. There are schools for the deaf which specialise in educating the most severely and multiply handicapped child through to those which cater for children with above-average abilities, taking pupils through public examinations and on to higher education.

Day Schools, Weekly Boarding and Full Boarding Schools

DAY SCHOOLS
Day Schools have the obvious advantage that children attending can live at home and be bused or taxied to the school. However, because of the low incidence of deafness such schools are likely to be small and with increased mainstreaming many such schools have closed. The travelling

can be a problem since children are often picked up in rotation and this can mean a very early start and a late return home for some. Depending on siting, the schools can develop links with mainstream schools but it should realised that only for a small number will the school be a neighbourhood school and therefore the contacts will not necessarily be the social contacts available near home. Where children are transported daily it can be difficult for the school to organise a strong out-of-school programme.

WEEKLY BOARDING

These schools still have to be reasonably close, but the weekends at home do allow the child to maintain home links. Such schools can have a well developed weekday extra-curricular activities programme allowing classmates to meet, socialise and play together.

FULL BOARDING SCHOOLS

Such schools tend to cater for children with very special needs. In today's educational climate they are almost certainly offering full board because the children who are sent to benefit from their special facilities frequently come from very distant homes. They cater for a variety of needs including taking children from very difficult backgrounds and also providing for children who, because of the severity and multiplicity of their handicaps, require 24-hour care.

Problems of Size and Distance

There are special schools which use sign language as a medium of instruction through to schools which use an entirely oral/aural approach. However, in reality these options are not *all* available to *all* pupils since hearing impaired children are few in number and geographically widely spread. Some, of course, are boarding schools but very long distances can certainly be a problem for parents to consider. This is a special problem for the Mary Hare Grammar School which draws able children from all over the United Kingdom, and also for some of the schools which have specialist facilities for deaf children with other disabilities such as visual impairment. Thankfully, multiple disabilities involving hearing impairment are relatively rare but the corollary is that provision is available in only a small number of places.

Where children do attend schools many miles away from their home, parents need to be clear that problems of contact have been carefully considered by the school and that efforts are being made to offset the recognised problems.

We have written elsewhere of the problems for special schools of increased mainstreaming, fewer deaf children because of the decline in the birthrate and because of improved medical care in the neo-natal period, but we should mention here that small numbers in schools create very serious problems for the curriculum. Small numbers of children can mean reduced staffing and therefore an inability to deliver a broad curriculum. They can also greatly reduce the possibility that children will be taught specialist subjects by specialist teachers. With the National Curriculum new demands are being placed upon some special schools which previously offered a narrower curriculum. Now all local authority maintained schools must follow the National Curriculum. Non-maintained and independent special schools will, we feel sure, all be endeavouring to meet the requirements of the National Curriculum or local authorities will withdraw their support for them, since the great majority of children in such schools are local authority funded.

Advantages of the Special School

Earlier in this chapter we concentrated on the advantages of the mainstream school as the placement for the hearing impaired child, but it is true to say that there are also advantages in the special school. A key advantage is its concentration of specially trained staff. It is most important that teachers have professional colleagues with whom they can share ideas and this is easily facilitated in the special school. Staff have to work much harder to achieve it in the partially hearing unit or as a support teacher in the mainstream. It is also easier to concentrate specialist equipment within the special school and easier to provide the services of technicians and specialist audiologists. In addition many special schools now have their own speech therapist and some have their own psychologist.

Another key advantage of the special school is in its small classes. This can be matched in the non-integrating unit but certainly not in the mainstream. Indeed the non-integrating unit has few advantages other than small classes and a relatively stress-free environment. Of course the special school is a protected environment but many are building close links with the unprotected outside world. A key to their success, after many have closed in recent years, is their ability to focus in specialist directions, providing service where local authorities would find it very difficult to provide a cost-effective alternative.

Visiting a Special School

It is very useful if those visiting the special school have a general idea of the level of deafness of the child they are considering placing there. This will not by itself allow you a comparison of degree of handicap but it will allow a comparison of degree of deafness. Degree of handicap depends on many other things including age at diagnosis, efficiency of amplification in the early years, intelligence, motivation and so on.

It is a good idea to observe children in the lower and upper part of the school. This should enable a visitor to make an approximate assessment of communication skills in the school. The best indicator of the success of any school is outcomes, so some attention must be paid to top groups in the school. We suggest visitors attempt to identify children's levels of expectation—where are they going from here—and how much at ease they are in communication. But remember, clarity of speech is neither a measure of intelligence nor the sole measure of success, so try to see as much of the children's work as possible.

In residential schools the bedrooms are obviously important and viewing them should allow you to assess whether any attempts are being made to create a homely atmosphere. It is also important to talk to care staff and ask about what goes on in the school in the evenings.

It is important to investigate the uncorrected written work of the children in various age groups throughout the school. Look at text books to see if they are modern, but mainly to see if they relate to the sort of books being used by normally hearing children of the same age.

Note the number of pupils in the school and try to assess whether there are sufficient children to allow careful grading and planning of courses and whether, particularly at secondary stage, there are sufficient pupils to allow for teaching specialist subjects. A guideline for minimum numbers at primary and secondary age might be 60 and 120 respectively, but remember if the school has forged strong links with neighbouring schools or colleges in order to draw on their resources, then smaller numbers may not be as serious a problem as it would be if the school were an entirely separate entity.

Time spent talking to the Head will enable the visitor to get a feel for the philosophy of the school (also read any available documents) and then the visitor should listen carefully to what is said by teachers and others around the school to assess whether the same philosophy is shared by the rest of the school.

Look at the use of hearing aids in every situation, the playground as well as the classrooms, and ask whether the school uses group hearing aids and radio aids and if so, in what situations. We believe that in a special school for severely and profoundly hearing impaired children there is an opportunity to exploit the superior output and frequency response characteristics of the group aid since the classes will be small. Radio aids can then be set aside for use on field study trips or other outside visits.

We think it is best not to pass too many comments but to listen carefully whilst viewing the school. Treat it as an opportunity to *look, listen and question*. After a visit is made by parents we would suggest a family discussion about whether it is felt that the child in question might fit into such an establishment.

Special School and the National Curriculum

We believe that parents can rest assured that all special schools will be doing their utmost to follow the National Curriculum and certainly for some it will mean that they will be being forced into following a broader curriculum than formerly. LEA schools will be following it because they are forced to by law and non-maintained schools (these are schools not supported by a single local authority but where the great majority of the children are funded by the LEA) will be following it because they realise that if they do not then LEAs will not send them children. We actually think that the great majority of schools believe the National Curriculum is a positive move and, provided it does not kill off teachers with the workload of testing and assessment (remember that the GCSE has drastically increased the testing and assessment load of teachers too), it has something positive to deliver to hearing impaired children. It can do much to raise expectations of what children should achieve. Just like normally-hearing children hearing impaired children will be being tested on their achievements at seven, eleven, fourteen and sixteen except where at sixteen they are being tested for GCSE.

Natural Aural Approaches (Non-Selective)

Around the country there are a few natural aural non-selective schools. They aim to cater for pupils who they believe can benefit from this wholly oral/aural approach to education. They believe that these children can thrive in classrooms where spoken language is the means of communication and sign language is not used. They are catering for mixed abilities on the understanding that the level of intelligence is not closely correlated with the child's ability to develop spoken language and knowing that it is only natural oral interaction which further develops the pupils' existing spoken language base.

In general they try to provide an approach to education which mirrors the mainstream, but adds the benefits of specialist teaching, high quality audiological support (since this approach definitely does not work without it) and small classes which allow much adult/child interaction in good acoustic conditions. If you are considering a school with a natural aural philosophy it is important to ask about the school's approach to the care and use of hearing aids, how frequently they are tested, what happens if aids break down, whether group hearing aids are used, whether radio aids are used for field trips, and so on. It is also important to enquire about the approaches to and opportunities for conversational work with the pupils.

Without exception the natural aural schools have high expectations of their children and in all the secondary schools attempts are made to enable the pupils to follow state examination courses. Obviously the ultimate goal of such schools is the integration of their pupils into the wider society.There are now numerous examples of severely and profoundly hearing impaired young people, former pupils of these schools, holding down good jobs and living a normal life within hearing society.

The natural aural schools follow a broad curriculum aiming to give the pupils experience in academic practical and creative areas. This makes them well placed to offer a full National Curriculum programme (something you should definitely ask about), which is, after all, only a broad curriculum within a national framework. Only time will tell us whether the testing and assessment within the National Curriculum will create too tight a strait-jacket for the curriculum and overburdening paperwork for the teachers, but it is already evident that the Government realise this danger since they have decided to test only English, Maths and Science at seven and eleven years, whereas earlier they had planned formal testing right across the curriculum.

All the schools using a natural aural approach participate fully in the affairs of the National Aural Group (NAG) which facilitates a considerable amount of professional contact and cross-fertilisation of ideas. The NAG can advise readers which schools follow the approach.

Natural Aural Approaches (Selective)

There is one grammar school for deaf children in the United Kingdom, the Mary Hare Grammar School at Newbury in Berkshire. (This corresponds to the one selective secondary school for the blind—New College, Worcester.) Mary Hare School has a national catchment area currently having pupils from more than eighty LEAs including Northern Ireland. The school believes that severely and profoundly hearing impaired children, who are academically able, have special educational needs which are not always capable of being met in the mainstream and selects its entry by examination, reports and interviews. The pupils then follow a full secondary programme to GCSE and A-Level with an oral/aural approach. All subjects are taught by specialist subject teachers who are also teachers of the deaf. The class groups are small and the subject spread very wide indeed. In recent years more than twenty subjects have been offered at GCSE with most being open for continuing to A-Level. The subject list includes French. Many former students of Mary Hare School are university graduates, some pursuing research to PhDs.

Burwood Park School, a selective secondary school with a technical bias, formerly had a joint examination procedure with the Mary Hare Grammar School, but with the advent of the National Curriculum and the need for all secondary schools to deliver this curriculum, including its technology components, the schools have gone their separate ways. It had long been questionable whether Burwood Park delivered a different curriculum for a different group of pupils other than that they took only boys.

Total Communication Approaches

It is highly likely that the curriculum aims of the schools using the total communication (TC) approach will be somewhat similar to those offering natural aural approaches, even more so now that the National Curriculum is prescribing the central subjects of the curriculum. Observers of TC approaches are often struck by its amorphous nature and find it difficult to be sure, precisely, what approach a particular school is offering. There are dangers that the TC school may become just a signing school, since there is great variability in the emphasis placed on the use of residual hearing. All the descriptions we have seen of TC include the importance of using residual hearing and also that TC is only adding something to the oral/aural approach. If the claims of TC are substantiated then the speech and language of children from such schools would be in advance of those from schools using other approaches, but this evidence is not forthcoming. Indeed research from the USA suggests that the opposite is the case. It has highlighted the paucity of English language usage from TC environments. Anyone considering a TC option for a child would need to satisfy themselves that TC really offers an advantage and should be aware that one UK school offering the approach is now planning to abandon it in favour of a move to using purely sign language as the first language.

We believe that people considering TC options for hearing impaired children need to question the long-term objectives for that child. Then, just as we have suggested lines of questioning for parents to use on a visit to a natural aural school, so some questions should be asked of a TC school. For example:

1 Are they preparing the child for wider society or for deaf society? If it is the former then spoken and written English is crucial to the child's development.
2 As before, what are the standards of children leaving the school? Look at writing and listen to spoken English. Also, what state examinations (GCSEs) are taken at the school and what grades are achieved? If it is a secondary school, how many pupils proceed to further and particularly higher education?
3 Clearly in a TC school signing skills are important. How well trained are the teachers in signing? Do they reach

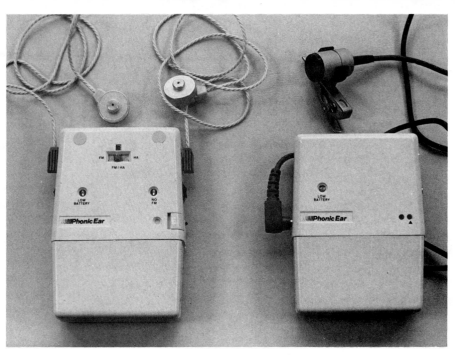

X A Type 1 radio system.

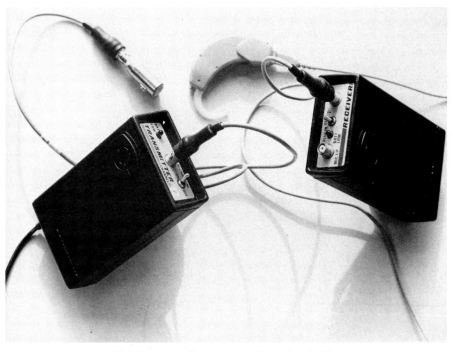

XI A Type 2 radio system with ear-level aid.

XII An Infra-Red system.

Council for the Advancement of Communication with Deaf People Stage 3 or better? Are parents trained and are ancillary staff at the school also trained—e.g., when meals are being served to children at lunch-time can the kitchen staff communicate with the children? And what about the school secretary, can she sign to children who have a problem and need to go to the school office? Our own experience is that such people are important elements in furthering and extending the language skills of children.

4 If input to the school from deaf people is regarded as important then are these also trained teachers?

5 What does the sign part of the TC consist of? Is it SE? Or is it SSE? Is it Paget Gorman? Is it a mixture of the aforementioned and BSL? Bear in mind that the latter is a language in its own right and not related to English.

Maternal Reflective Approach

There is only one all-age school in the United Kingdom using the maternal reflective approach originally devised at St Michielsgestel, Holland, by Father Van Uden. However, the approach is used in some areas of the country outside the special school.

REGULAR REVIEWS

Whether children are in a special school for hearing impaired children or in the mainstream it is important that as well as continued educational monitoring they have a regular audiological review.

1 The hearing aids should be tested electro-acoustically and every six months, or at least annually, a review should be made of whether the aids are still appropriate. A monthly check should indicate if new earmoulds are required and if so fresh impressions can be taken.

2 There should be a monthly tympanometry check to

monitor the condition of the child's middle ear.Work we have done has shown that in addition to the sensori-neural deafness that the children have they are just as likely as any other child to suffer from middle-ear problems which would, in their case, add to an already serious hearing problem. Every service for hearing impaired children should have a direct line of referral for such children to an otologist.

3 Six-monthly, or at least annually, the children should have a complete audiological review. This should include pure-tone testing by air and bone, with masking if necessary, tympanometry and stapedius reflex tests, and speech tests of hearing of the sort that the child can manage. There should be a check of amplification requirements. We think it is well worth keeping a cumulative audiogram to ensure that any deterioration (or improvement) in hearing level is immediately spotted.

* * *

It is hoped that the information presented in this chapter will better inform non-specialists of the range of educational opportunities available for hearing impaired children, but there is no adequate substitute for visits and asking the right questions.

References

1 Bown, E., 'Attitudes to the placement of pre-school hearing impaired children in normal nurseries', M. Ed. Dissertation, University of Manchester, 1981.

2 Powers. S., 'A survey of units for hearing impaired children', Part 1, *J. Brit. Assn. Teachers of the Deaf*, 14, 3, (1990), pp. 61-79.

5 Educational Placement

Historically it seems that the educational placement of hearing impaired children has been dictated more by the available educational provision than by the real needs of the children that the provision is meant to serve. We are sure that a sensory handicap such as deafness merits a *range* of provision. This is vital because the educational and social impact of the disability can range from very slight at one end of the spectrum to very severe at the other.

This small volume is not intended to be a text book on history but knowledge of where education of the deaf has been and inklings of where it may be going are important for those with a hearing impaired child in their care. Parents will have important decisions to make about their children's education at various points and the information below could help them to understand the 'scene': their rights and responsibilities and the duties of the local education authorities.

Legislation in 1893 ensured the availability of special education for all deaf and blind children and the early twentieth century saw the rapid development of special schools and a later and more gradual development of special classes in ordinary schools (Salford 1948). These became known as *partially hearing units* and were originally intended for remedial work with children with less severe problems than those requiring education in a special school. However, the dominating feature of education of the deaf in the early years was the special school, either day or residential, where specialist skills and knowledge were built up and brought to bear on the educational problems of the deaf.

Parallel developments were taking place in audiology, a new discipline gathering knowledge about deafness, its causation, detection, its medical and surgical treatment and its remedy with increasingly powerful hearing aids. Pioneers such as Alexander Ewing and Thomas Watson at Manchester

University were defining the areas of interest for the educational audiologist. Watson wrote:

> The function of the educational audiologist should be to enable a hearing impaired child to obtain early and high quality listening experiences and to provide his parents with the support and knowledge that will enable them to ensure his optimal psychological, social and linguistic development.

Clearly the 1944 Education Act was a landmark in the education of the handicapped in this country since it laid down the ground rules for local education authorities with respect to special education:

> . . . to afford for all pupils opportunities for education offering such variety of instruction and training as may be desirable in view of their different ages, abilities and aptitudes, and of the different periods which they may be expected to remain at school . . .

Local authorities were required to identify all those requiring special education and to ensure that adequate provision was made for them. Following the 1944 Act the Ministry of Education published a booklet in 1946 defining handicap within 11 categories, the categories ascertained by medical officers. (There was thus a powerful medical input to an educational area.) *Deaf* and *partially deaf* were two separate categories. Thus began a period of expansion in special education, mostly in special schools. Existing schools flourished and new ones opened, even residential special schools for the partially deaf.

Improved methods of detection meant that the numbers of children with partial deafness increased (many previously had been hidden amongst the 'slow learners' or maladjusted groups) and along with it the number of partially hearing units rose from two in 1948 to 212 in 1971 and over 500 now. Initially the partially hearing units, although placed in mainstream schools, remained very separate from those schools and little time would be spent by the children in mainstream classes, this in spite of the fact that generally the children had only moderate hearing losses. This has changed in recent years with many hearing impaired children returning to their unit base for support work for only a few periods in the week. It is now perhaps even more difficult to generalise because more of the children with moderate losses are completely integrated into ordinary classrooms and the units are accepting more profoundly impaired children who require increased support work.

In 1962, as a result of pressure to view handicapped children more positively, legislation changed the term 'partially deaf' to 'partially hearing' and severely and profoundly impaired children were no longer excluded from ordinary schools.

Throughout the Sixties and Seventies there were positive moves towards the education of the partially hearing within ordinary primary and secondary schools, either in the special units mentioned above or by integration into ordinary classes with support from visiting teachers of the deaf. Table 2 shows the increase in the number of teachers supporting children in the mainstream. It has been argued by many people that this development could be attributed to the progressive outlook of teachers of the deaf and pressure group activity from parents rather than to the influence of government or legislation.

Table 2

Teachers Supporting Children in Mainstream

1958	1969	1973	1975	1987
4	200	283	363	495

It has always been difficult to give precise numbers of children in particular educational environments because of the different ways in which they are classified by local education authorities and also because of the different ways in which the statistics are collected. However, in a very recent survey carried out for the British Association of Teachers of the Deaf[1] the educational whereabouts of UK hearing impaired children is clearly shown and indicates that the overwhelming majority of hearing impaired children are educated in the mainstream (see Table 3).

Table 3

The Educational Placement of Pre-school and
School-aged Children

Source	England and Wales	Scotland
Schools for the Deaf/PH	2354	130
Units	2263	95
Pre-School	1721	133
Mainstream Schools	6689	648
Other Special Schools	1625	43
Notified to Service		
a) Variable conductive loss	28486	152
b) Severe monaural loss	2815	37
Mainstream without hearing aids	9895	509
Totals	55848	1747

Perhaps of even more interest is the place where teachers of the deaf are employed. In 1978 41 per cent were working in special schools.[2] By 1988 this had fallen to 30.6 per cent.[1]

THE WARNOCK REPORT

It can be safely said that teachers of the deaf looked forward to the outcome of the investigations into special education of the *Warnock Committee*. This report was published in 1978. The report made many recommendations (228), the key thrust being in three areas: pre-school education, tertiary education and teacher training. Interestingly these were areas where much progress had already been made in deaf education since it was in deaf education that pre-school parent guidance had been prominent and it had long been established that teachers of the deaf (and blind) must hold specialist advanced qualifications in order to hold posts teaching this group of sensorily handicapped children.

The report also proposed the abolition of categories of handicapped children and young people and promoted the concept of considering children's special educational needs and seeking to integrate them into mainstream provision wherever it would not be to their disadvantage. The scope of the ensuing Education Act was heavily criticised by Mary Warnock, leaders in special education, teachers' associations and the educational press. Reeves, in the *Journal of the British Association of Teachers of the Deaf,* said that what many had hoped would provide a charter for children in need turned out to be 'more of an administrators' delight. The Act put its emphasis on assessments, reviews, appeals, and such like, and said very little about educational principles and practice covered in the Warnock Report.

THE 1981 EDUCATION ACT

The 1981 Education Act, fully implemented by April 1983, recognised the Warnock recommendation and abolished the categories of handicap established by the Ministry of Education in 1946. Medical descriptions of the children's disabilities were replaced by a 'statement' of their special educational needs. Local authorities were given the responsibility of identifying those children whose needs required special educational provision.

The Act established the principle that children with special educational needs should be educated in ordinary schools:

> . . . so far as is reasonably practicable, and are to associate in the activities of the school with the other children. This principle is subject to account having been taken of the views of parents, the ability of the school to meet the child's special educational needs, consistency

with the provision of efficient education for other children in the school and the efficient use of resources by the local education authority.

In theory there was thus an onus on the local authority to assess the child's needs independently of the available resources or provision. There is no doubt though that, because the Government did not provide additional resources to implement the Act, some assessments were, and still are, geared to the available provision. This has been highlighted by a recent DES circular which has drawn attention to the undesirability of resource-led statementing by LEAs. Many local authorities have also found it necessary to employ additional administrative staff and educational psychologists while at the same time cutting back on the number of teachers. In a recent survey of 69 local authorities the average statementing time was 21 months. In other words, if a child is coming towards a key decision-time parents are to be strongly advised to start the assessment process very early. Another local authority ploy has been to mainstream hearing-handicapped children and then say that because they are in the mainstream they do not require a statement. The authors know of many children with very severe hearing losses who are not statemented. This is fine while (or if) things are going well, but when things go wrong and the parents perceive that their child is not getting the help needed, they then realise they have no comeback on an authority which is not providing help—because they do not agree that such help should be provided in the context of a statement of need. In our view there are more potential benefits to the parent and child of a statement being drawn up than not, and every child with a significant hearing loss should have one.

Although the Secretary of State for Education and Science 'expects that statements should be processed within six months and that only in exceptional circumstances should it take longer than this' in practice this is clearly not happening and the advice to parents must be to get the statementing process under way as well in advance as possible of key points in the child's educational career. Once a statement of special need has been made it should be reviewed every year.

A Parents' Charter?

Section 4 of the Education Act 1981 places local education authorities under a duty to identify special needs and, where appropriate, to prepare a statement. We might ask the question, 'Why was it suggested that the new Act was a parents' charter?'

1 Parents can request an assessment of need from the local authority, and the Secretary of State has let it be known that sympathy will be shown to the parents' case in any dispute.
2 Parents have the right to be present at any assessment of their child.
3 Parents have the right to receive information and to be consulted. For example, parents must be informed of the LEA's intention to make an assessment of their child.
4 They can put forward their views during the assessment period.
5 They have the right to receive copies of information and advice produced during the statementing process.
6 They can comment on the draft statement.
7 They can appeal against the local authority's conclusions on the special provisions required by the child. (This is heard by a local appeals tribunal which can be overturned by the local authority—the parents' only recourse then is to appeal to the Secretary of State. The whole appeals procedure can take more than a year and cause a great deal of stress to parents.

It has been argued by some educationists that special education services are dominated by the needs of the mentally, emotionally or physically handicapped and that strategies appropriate for them are imposed on the minority categories of the deaf and the blind. The 1981 Education Act has strengthened this feeling since many authorities have planned a generic service for special needs. By the law of averages these services have been headed by staff from the mentally handicapped/physically handicapped areas who, traditionally, have little knowledge of the normally intelligent, but sensorily handicapped child for whom very different teaching approaches are appropriate. We believe that this is part of what we said above, that the Act was an administrator's delight. We know of many services where prior to the Act there was a Head of the Service for Hearing Impaired Children who held the support work together, fought for resources for the deaf in a tight budgetary scene, provided specialist services such as educational audiology on an area or county basis, but who has now been replaced by a generic special-needs person who knows very little about deafness and its requirements in terms of support. In our view this is bad news for parents and for hearing impaired children and it means that parents now have to be even more vigilant in setting out the case for the provision of support for the special educational needs of their children.

An example of this is the question of the special school for hearing impaired children. The figures given above show the very small percentage, less than five per cent, of deaf children who are being educated separately from their hearing peers in a special school. We entirely support the fact that this should be the case with the great majority of hearing impaired children, but there are some local authorities whose administrators appear only to have read the section of the Act which says that 'all children with special educational needs should be educated in ordinary schools' without reading any of the provisos or the Warnock Report reservations (Department of Education and Science, 1978, p. 121), which said that special schools should continue to feature prominently *in the range* of provision for children with special educational needs. As Reeves said, most people seem to appreciate the need for the severely mentally, emotionally and physically handicapped to have a special school option but too many seem to believe that children with a sensory problem do not experience any substantial difficulties provided they are equipped with appropriate aids.

Traditionally the country has catered for about two per cent of children in special schools yet Warnock suggested that there may be as many as 18 or 20 per cent of children who actually require special education of some kind at some point in their educational career. What seems to us to be crucial is that we monitor this potential need at key points and, from widely based provision, allocate resources according to children's needs.

The deaf are certainly vulnerable since it is not always realised that in addition to their peripheral sensory and communication problems there may also be cognitive difficulties which can constitute a severe learning difficulty. The other problem is, of course, that mainstreaming is seen by some as a cheaper alternative to special schools. When this is the case deaf children may be left in environmentally hostile situations unmonitored and unsupported. This can be good neither educationally nor socially.

So how do educators and parents operate in this most difficult of decision-making areas? In America the concept of 'least restrictive environment' originated in an education Bill (PL 94-142) which described a situation where children would have the maximum opportunity for participation in ordinary educational procedures. Many people thought this meant only 'mainstreaming' as they did in the United Kingdom when the Education Act established the principle that children with special educational needs should be educated in ordinary schools. That seems pretty clear but many people missed reading the qualifying phrase (or took no notice of it)—'so far as is reasonable . . .'—mentioned above.

TYPES OF MAINSTREAM PROVISION

The practice of educating hearing impaired children alongside their hearing peers is well established in Britain and the USA. In fact Britain mainstreams more children (52.1%) with hearing losses greater than 50dB than any other European country, with Denmark (43.8%), Italy (50.1%) and Ireland

(34.5%) being the other countries mainstreaming relatively large numbers of children.

There are many types of provision which might come under the heading of 'mainstreamed provision'. Certainly parents must ask the question, 'How much interaction with normally hearing children will this provision give my child?' Some of the main variants of mainstreaming are listed below:

1 Complete integration or mainstreaming within the ordinary class without any supportive help.
2 Mainstreaming with varying levels of classroom-based individual support.
3 Basing the children in a resource room or base unit and integrating them on a part-time basis into the ordinary class. The subjects they integrate for can also vary.
4 Team teaching by an ordinary teacher and a specialist teacher of the deaf to an integrated class into which is placed one or more hearing impaired children.
5 Reversed mainstreaming, where normally hearing pupils become part of a class of hearing impaired pupils. This is less common in the United Kingdom, but seems to be done more frequently at the nursery end where the educators of the hearing impaired rate very highly, perhaps more highly than elsewhere, the influence of ordinary children. Certainly special schools for the hearing impaired have set up nurseries for deaf children and have then sought to bring in normally hearing children to interact with them. However, by far the greatest number of deaf children have any nursery education they may get in an ordinary nursery, perhaps with the support of a visiting teacher of the deaf.
6 Self-contained classes or units from which the pupils go to ordinary classes for one or more specific academic subjects.
7 Completely self-contained classes or units with little or no contact with normally hearing peers.

The mainstreaming may be into state-maintained schools, selective or comprehensive schools at secondary age and in a few cases into independent schools, either paid for by the local education authority with specialist support provided by the LEA or completely unsupported.

Another option suggested by American writers is to put a qualified teacher of the deaf in charge of a class of normally hearing children into which one or more hearing impaired children are integrated. This could have benefits, although we have not heard of it being carried out in the United Kingdom. An even more important development would be to ensure that every mainstream teacher had appropriate in-service training if hearing impaired children were being placed in their classes. This is clearly not happening and more will be said about this later.

AREAS TO LOOK AT WHEN CONSIDERING EDUCATIONAL PLACEMENT

The educational problems of the deaf have never been simple to assess and we believe that there are some key questions that need to be addressed when decisions are being made about placement. They are especially important in relation to very severely hearing impaired children. Remember fewer than five per cent of hearing impaired children are currently in special schools and they on average, though not in all cases, will be the deafest children and/or children with handicaps additional to deafness. One needs to consider how deaf the child is and be aware of the environmental conditions likely to be faced by children in different types of educational placement. Then one can consider intellectual and developmental factors in the child. Parents must be involved in activating and participating in the decision-making process leading up to the placement of their child.

It is our opinion that the hearing impaired population is so lacking in homogeneity that there is a need for a wide variety of educational provision. Selection for that provision should be led by the child's individual special educational needs and not governed solely by cost or what provision is currently available in a particular local authority. Sensory deafness is a relatively rare disability and we see it as advantageous for local authorities to share provision where they have insufficient children to warrant making a particular form of provision for themselves. This may well be the only way that a whole variety of approaches can be truly made available to hearing impaired children. A cascade approach ranging from total integration into mainstream with and without support, through units and 'resource bases' to day and residential special schools would seem to be ideal. Whilst consistency is important there should be opportunity for movement through the cascade and this could relate to annual reviews of the child's Statement of Special Educational Need.

Considering Mainstreaming

We shall consider mainstreaming—the placing of the hearing impaired child in an ordinary class for some or all of his education—in more practical detail later but at the moment we want to mention some of the pre-placement factors which should be considered.

SCHOOL RELATED FACTORS

There are many factors within the school's structure and organisation which can affect the desirability of placing there a sensorily handicapped child. None of them have overriding weight but together they may indicate or contra-indicate the desirability of going ahead with the placement. Lynas (1986)[3] has outlined some of the significant dimensions along which schools vary:

1 Size—some schools cater for over two thousand pupils, others for less than a hundred.
2 Organisation—there are many ways of organising teaching groups within a school, for example, vertical groupings (when more than one age group is in one class) team teaching, streaming by ability, subject teaching, and so on.
3 Buildings—these vary a great deal in their shape, size, layout, for example open plan or separate classrooms and

single storey or multi-storey buildings. Open-plan classrooms can dramatically increase background noise levels if inadequately sound treated, and multi-storey buildings can provide much increased structure-borne noise to affect the hearing impaired child's ability to hear 'messages' from the teacher.

4 School philosophy—schools differ in their ethos, for example in the emphasis they place on certain aims, firm discipline, high educational standards, individual care and all-round development.

5 Atmosphere—schools can have a range of noticeable atmospheres such as friendly, intimate, purposeful, industrious, casual, laissez-faire, authoritarian—anarchic!

6 Different levels of noise are present in schools according to the prevailing acoustic conditions, but also according to teaching style and to the level of pupil noise which will be tolerated by the teachers.

We need to consider very carefully the sort of educational environment which would be most suitable for particular hearing impaired children. For example, high levels of noise have been shown by many researchers to greatly affect the reception of speech through personal hearing aids. A school with many problem and difficult children may well find it difficult to integrate a hearing impaired child and a small friendly caring environment may, for a particular child, be better than a large diffuse comprehensive school. So clearly those responsible for placement must look in some detail at the *particular school* into which there is a possibility of placing a hearing impaired child. School features as well as child features *must* be considered before the child is placed, not when things start to go wrong later after a bad placement decision. Poor placement decisions may be avoided if the Statement of Special Educational Need includes specific references, for example to small classes, or the level of individual support needed.

Teachers and Teaching Style

The hearing impaired child needs to interact with the teacher and other children in a great variety of situations and these situations are not equally difficult. For example, the child may find it much easier to follow when engaged in an activity with a few other children and the teacher around a small table than when the class is being treated as one large group. In general hearing impaired children follow better when they are being interacted with individually or in small groups, but of course they also benefit from the stimulation of other children. However, this can be counterbalanced if classroom group work results in an increase in ambient noise levels. Where this happens, the problems of the deaf child are increased, and for this reason many say they find a didactic whole-class approach easier to follow. This is perhaps a question of teacher education rather than child education.

In small-group co-operative projects the hearing impaired child can benefit greatly from the help of other children. Co-operation and sharing and being part of a team are important skills for the child to learn. This works especially well if the child has the opportunity both to be led and to lead the group. How well this area is handled can help decide whether the child is integrated into or isolated from the class.

We must also be aware that teachers vary enormously in other aspects of their teaching style, for example rate of speaking, clarity and manner of presentation. Teachers vary in the amount they talk before they check that the children have understood. They also vary in how they actually check understanding. Those with experience in education of the hearing impaired are well aware of the 'head-nodding syndrome' where the child nods 'yes' when asked if he understands—many children do this for years while falling farther and farther behind in their learning. Teachers also vary in the way they summarise the main points of a lesson for the child and the amount they use written back-up material to reinforce learning and to provide clear guidelines for revision. They also vary in how they react to verbal contributions in the lesson from the child.

Hearing impaired children are greatly helped by careful use of the blackboard (i.e. not talking whilst facing away from the children and making careful summaries of the main points of a lesson); even better is the use of an overhead projector. Teachers can help by reformulating questions to give more clues and particularly by using the reflection technique where the teacher repeats the answer of another pupil so that the hearing impaired child can hear, aided possibly by a radio transmitter, the correct, (or incorrect!) answer.

Lynas (1986)[3] has looked at the way that teachers in the ordinary class react to having a hearing impaired child in their class. It seems that there is a continuum of positive discrimination. First, there is *none at all* i.e. the child is accepted if he can cope with only a 'normal' amount of attention. Then there is *limited positive discrimination,* where the teacher sees the hearing impaired child as only one of a variety of children with special needs, for example the slow learners or those with reading difficulties. They would not offer specialised help but would be willing to make minor adjustments to teaching technique such as facing the child when speaking and seating them in an advantageous position in class. At the next level the teacher offers *considerable positive discrimination,* where the teacher makes carefully thought-out changes to teaching style to help the hearing impaired child. This might include adjusting speaking rate and articulation in order to improve clarity, using the blackboard or overhead projector to clarify terms or provide summaries of the work covered. The teacher will ensure that the hearing impaired child sits in a good position, and uses reflection techniques and checks to ensure understanding. There is no doubt that some become so skilled that they anticipate problems and pre-empt them by preparatory work. At the other end of the continuum there is *excessive positive discrimination,* where the teacher goes overboard making concessions to the hearing impaired child at the expense of the other children, gives him a much bigger share of individual time, praises effusively only modest achievements and quite frankly risks alienating the whole class against this privileged child. Giving more help than is actually needed does the child a disservice. Other children in particular come to resent such over-support, and view it as an intrusion.

Clearly, apart from the last level, all of the levels on the continuum could be useful to a hearing impaired child providing it was the right child for the particular level of discrimination and providing that any shortfall in input could be made up by a specialist teacher of the deaf.

Pros and Cons of Integrated Provision

The advantages of integrated provision are quite well rehearsed in the consciousness of educators and of parents too, with home base, a broad educational curriculum, exposure to a normal speech and language environment, social contact and social adjustment featuring very highly in people's thinking. This is rightly so and we have spoken and written about these advantages over separate special and possibly residential provision. Knowledge of the effects of institutionalisation is much greater now, but the risks are still there and steps have to be taken to ensure that children do not become socially handicapped in order to prevent them becoming educationally handicapped, and deafness is essentially a social handicap. There is no doubt also that even some special schools have failed to deliver the educational goods with a restricted curriculum and low aspirations for the children. While some such schools are still to be found, happily most are now part of educational history. The aforementioned features in favour of mainstreaming are very powerful and in fact overpowering for the great majority of hearing impaired children who should, quite rightly, be mainstreamed. However, such placement should be appropriate for the particular child and some arguments against mainstreaming should also be considered before placement is finally decided.

Such a placement *can* put too much pressure on the pupil having to cope with large classes, poor acoustic conditions and less individual help from a specialist teacher of the deaf. It can, unless pupils are very carefully selected and given adequate support, result in pupils being isolated from the hearing children in the class as well as being segregated from other children with hearing problems. It is not uncommon to find that even where hearing impaired children are not actively discriminated against they are not 'chosen' as best friend. Children in single-teacher units can be especially vulnerable to staff changes and again it is not uncommon when a teacher leaves for there to be a period when there is no specialist teacher at all to help hearing impaired children. Such children are also specially vulnerable if the teacher is poor since it is not uncommon for hearing impaired children in such units to be taught for several years by the same teacher. It is also disadvantageous—because of the small numbers of hearing impaired children—for them to be taught in wide vertical age groups. The teachers of the deaf themselves, because of their position as possibly the only teacher of the deaf in a mainstream school, can become isolated from professional support. Mainstreaming can be regarded as a cheaper option by local authorities and prevent out-county/authority placements in special schools.

Parents would be well advised to ask to see as wide a variety of options for their child as possible and they should not be frightened of asking searching questions of each establishment they visit.

Successful Integration
Successful integration seems to happen when the following conditions are met.

1 The child is not too far (perhaps no more than eighteen months) behind his mainstream peers, e.g. in language and maths areas.
2 The child has an outgoing personality.
3 The child's auditory skills plus lip-reading are good.
4 The child has specialist support according to his needs.
5 The child has excellent audiological back-up and personal equipment including radio aids.
6 Intelligence and degree of hearing loss have not been shown to have a *major* influence on mainstreaming success

except towards the outer edges of high and low. The major criterion is the use the child has made of residual hearing. The deafer the child is, though, the more he or she would be dependent on the small amount of residual hearing and on lip-reading skills, and would suffer seriously in adverse noise conditions, particularly without specialist amplification systems.

7 The mainstream teacher/teachers are warm and accepting of the child and willing to take advice on how to help and put effort into providing extra attention.

8 Last but not least—very supportive parents.

There is no doubt that out in the mainstream there is a new generation of children who are handicapped by deafness but who have been diagnosed early, well fitted with hearing aids and have developed the level of communication skills which enables them to hold their own with normally hearing children. However, there are special children who, because of some feature—be it high or very low intelligence, or additionally handicapping conditions—whom we feel are better placed in educational environments which can better cater for their special educational needs. The decisions for professionals and parents are extremely difficult since it is always going to be debatable what level of retardation would preclude the mainstreaming of the child on educational grounds.

Social advantages of integration cannot be fulfilled if the child is effectively isolated from hearing peers by the level of the handicap. Such a child will also be unable to access the curriculum and be under increasing pressure of not following what is going on in the classroom. We certainly have evidence of hearing impaired children 'opting out' not necessarily disruptively, but quietly letting the curriculum wash over them. An example of a mainstreamed very severely hearing impaired child we saw recently serves to highlight this problem. She had done very well in the primary school and the educational 'slippage' at secondary was very gradual, but by the fourth form she was reduced to studying only English,

Mathematics, General Science and Computer Studies. The school and parents had perceived these as the subjects the girl was 'best' at but they could well have been the only subjects which she had managed to access or which she was being forced to do (for example, her English was also poor). What a narrow curriculum for an above averagely intelligent girl—no History, Geography, Music and so on. This problem of a very restricted curriculum should happen less in the future because the National Curriculum demands that children follow a broad range of subjects and if a school were to 'disapply' a child from a particular subject, it would have to show what was being put in its place and that replacement would have to be justified.

References

1 BATOD, Report on Staffing and Salary Situation in Schools, *J. Brit Assn Teachers of the Deaf,* (13), 3, (1989), mag. p. 2.
2 BATOD, Report on Staffing and Salary Situation in Schools, *J. Brit Assn Teachers of the Deaf* (2), 3, (1978), mag. p. 10.
3 Lynas, W., *Integrating the Handicapped into Ordinary Schools—A Study of Hearing Impaired Pupils,* Croom Helm, London, 1986.

6 Hearing Impaired Children and the National Curriculum

The basic curriculum (what we teach and how we teach it) to be taught in Britain's schools has now been prescribed in law. As from September 1989 mainstream schools have been obliged to follow the National Curriculum, special schools following suit in September 1990. Previously what was taught in schools was largely up to the schools themselves, although in reality most schools, particularly at secondary level, were 'hooked' into an examination system that made the freedom to teach what they wished more apparent than real.

One of the things the National Curriculum responded to was the rapid expansion in subjects offered in secondary schools, an expansion of choice which enabled young people to opt out of studying, at a very early age, subjects that the Government believed to be essential subjects such as Mathematics and Geography. Also, the Government and the schools' inspectorate (HMI) perceived what they believed to be an unevenness in the educational standards being achieved around the country.

The Education Reform Act (1988) says that the curriculum should promote the spiritual, moral, cultural, mental and physical level of schoolchildren and of society at large. The National Curriculum aims to provide for all children a curriculum which is *broad,* encompassing a wide range of experience, *balanced,* giving subjects sufficient time on the curriculum to be effective, *relevant,* providing experiences which can lead to opportunities in adult life, and *differentiated,* matching the individual needs of children.

Schools are now bound by law to teach certain subjects to age 16 and over the next few years tests to assess whether children have achieved targets in those subjects will be introduced. There will be continual monitoring of progress but reported assessments must take place at or near the end of each 'key stage'. These will be at the ages of 7, 11, 14 and 16 years for most pupils. The Task Group on Assessment and Testing (TGAT) is currently preparing Standard Assessment Tasks (SATs), initially in the core subject areas of Mathematics, English and Science. Over the next few years this will extend to other subjects of the National Curriculum.

COMPOSITION OF THE NATIONAL CURRICULUM

The composition of the National Curriculum is as follows:

   *CORE SUBJECTS: English, Mathematics and Science
   *FOUNDATION SUBJECTS: Technology, History, Geography, Music, Art, Physical Education, Religious Education and at least one modern language.

   Local education authorities are required to deliver to children the National Curriculum within a broad and balanced curriculum. That is, the National Curriculum is not everything that will be taught to children, the Government accepting that there are study areas other than those on which they are legislating.

How Does This Affect the Handicapped?
It should be remembered that until the passing of the Education (Handicapped Children) Act in 1970, there was a very large group of children with severe learning disorders who had no right to education at all. The Warnock Report stressed that the goals of education were the same for all pupils, but it was not until the Education Reform Act that statute finally recognised the right of all handicapped children in the UK to have a broad, balanced and differentiated curriculum, relevant to their needs. We believe that this legislation providing 'entitlement' presents the possibilities of a real step forward for deaf children, but on all sides there has to be understanding and the will to deliver what has been

legislated for.

It is suggested in Curriculum Guidance 2, 'A Curriculum for All' (a National Curriculum Council publication), that there may well be slightly different emphases in mainstream schools and special schools. In *mainstream schools* it is clear that there is a broad curriculum but is it accessible to all pupils? Do all the staff know which children have special needs, the nature of their needs and how best to meet them? Can they ensure maximum access for special needs children? A key question relates to the availability and adequacy of resources, and support and training of staff. The schools will need to designate staff to co-ordinate school policy on special needs and to ensure that the progress of children is appropriately monitored and evaluated. There will also need to be regular revision of the schools' approaches in the light of experience of implementing the National Curriculum. Parents of hearing impaired children will need to discuss with staff the points generated above. The many government initiatives have produced a massive workload for staff in schools and the authors are aware of many schools that are so busy responding to other areas that they are not yet considering their responses to special needs children.

In *special schools* it is felt that in general, though by no means in all schools, the emphasis will be on extending the breadth of the curriculum. Here plans to implement the National Curriculum may well need to include curricular links with nearby ordinary schools providing an opportunity to extend a special school's subject range. This would also have the effect of producing a compatibility which would enable the hearing impaired child, if it was felt appropriate, to move back into the mainstream of education. Repeated surveys by the Schools Inspectorate have highlighted deficiencies in some special schools' provisions for science, design technology, home economics and music, amongst other subject areas, and clearly parents and those involved in placement decisions need to ask pointed questions about how special schools, and also mainstream services for hearing impaired children propose to meet the requirements of the National Curriculum in these areas.

It is likely that many teachers, particularly in primary schools, will feel that their expertise is weak in the science and technology areas. There must be resources put into ensuring that such teachers have an opportunity to strengthen skills in these vital areas. The problem is not likely to be so acute in secondary schools, with their wide use of specialisms, but even here these are national shortage subjects and many children are being taught by non-specialists simply because specialists cannot be recruited. Also, very small special schools are particularly vulnerable since it is unlikely that they will be able to afford the wide range of specialists necessary to deliver the National Curriculum at secondary level. However, a positive approach to these areas will show that a school sees the demands of the National Curriculum as a chance to broaden the opportunities for the hearing impaired child rather than as a series of externally imposed constraints which just add to the difficulties.

Wherever the child is placed we are sure that a question commonly asked by both parents and teachers is likely to be: 'Will hearing impaired children in general, or this child in particular, need to have some requirement of the National Curriculum modified or lifted altogether?' In answer, it seems that there will be no 'whole group' rules, i.e. hearing impaired children as a group will not be 'disapplied from' (taken out of) any of the National Curriculum requirements. We are very pleased that this is the case since it will make all those concerned with the child look at that child's individual specific special needs and any modification to or disapplication from a curriculum would relate to the particular child.

Any change to the National Curriculum will require a change in the pupil's Statement of Special Educational Needs and for current children local authorities have until 1990 to rewrite statements in the light of such demands. In those statements any changes to the requirements will need to be clearly shown and will have to indicate the reasons for change or disapplication along with an outline of how the pupil's entitlement to a broad and balanced curriculum is to be preserved. The onus is upon the local authority to detail the provision the child requires in terms of the facilities and equipment, staffing arrangements, methods and approaches and, wherever relevant, educational environment, access and transport provision. The above should be described in clear terms and not be vague. Also, since each statement must have an input from a teacher of the deaf, we see it as an opportunity for such teachers to specify what resources are required to deliver the curriculum to the child.

Under section 19 of the Education Reform Act headteachers may give directions making temporary exceptions for up to six months in the first instance from any or all of the National Curriculum requirements for individual pupils who are statemented. The situation is somewhat fluid at this stage but the Department of Education and Science does not expect that more than a small number of statements will need to be substantially revised since it expects schools to be planning for children to participate in the National Curriculum. Aspects of policy in this area are to be monitored and reviewed as a result of experience within local education authorities and schools. Of particular concern to us, and no doubt to parents too, are children without statements. There is very varied practice among local authorities and some do not statement any child who is receiving education in the mainstream. Some of these are very handicapped children who will undoubtedly require special arrangements when it comes to standard assessment tasks. Some professionals are already asking whether such children should be statemented to ensure that they get the help they need and that their mainstream teachers get the opportunity for the in-service training which *they* need.

ATTAINMENT TARGETS

Within each key stage there will be a series of attainment targets towards which children will work and on which they will be assessed. It is thought that, based on these assessments, teachers will plan what the child needs in the future. Such work is not new of course—it has always been the hallmark of good practice in education that teachers assess progress and plan the next steps. However, in the standard assessment tasks this becomes more formalised and it is assumed that where there are problems teachers will be able to use diagnostic materials to detect underlying difficulties when a child seems to be making little or no progress at a particular level.

Section 3 of the child's statement should contain detail of any modification or disapplication of the National Curriculum requirements and should include any programmes of study outside the National Curriculum framework specially designed to meet the child's needs, as well as any modifications needed to the attainment targets, the programmes of study or to the assessment and testing arrangements. If no modification or exemption is shown in section 3 then a maintained school is obliged to offer all of the subjects of the National Curriculum without modification for that pupil at a level appropriate to the pupil's ability, unless the provisions of the National Curriculum are excluded or modified by virtue of other provisions of the 1988 Act by a headteacher or by the Secretary of State.

As parents can appeal against the findings of the Statement of Special Educational Need so can they appeal against the modification or disapplication of all or part of the National Curriculum, firstly to a local appeals committee and finally to the Secretary of State. As attainment targets and programmes of study for each subject in the curriculum are published, annual reviews of a child's statement must be made and any required amendments made.

One area of the National Curriculum where many hearing impaired children will require a curriculum change will be the learning of a modern foreign language. In many special schools this has been excluded from the curriculum. In services for hearing impaired children in the mainstream this has traditionally been one area of the curriculum where hearing impaired children have been withdrawn in order to provide time for support work. For the great majority of deaf children we are convinced that this should not be the case and in the school at which one of us is Principal, eleven profoundly deaf children achieved the top grades (A-C) in the 1990 GCSE French examinations. The only concession in the examination was that in the listening test, rather than listening to a tape recording, the children listened to a teacher of French speaking. At all levels we are sure that children can gain great benefit from study of foreign language and foreign culture.

The question of withdrawal from the curriculum for support work is a thorny one—from what do you withdraw children when an increasing portion of the curriculum comes directly under statute? Also there is evidence in some schools that hearing impaired children have ended up with a very narrow curriculum because of withdrawal even though the host mainstream school has in fact a very broad curriculum. Clearly, achieving a balance between the needs of the children from the point of view of their linguistic handicap associated with deafness and their need for a broad curriculum as outlined in the National Curriculum will not be easy. There will need to be close liaison between teachers of the deaf and mainstream teachers to ensure that as much of the National Curriculum as possible is actually delivered to the child.

In partially hearing units decisions will need to be made about which subjects will be studied in the mainstream supported by teachers of the deaf, and which in the unit itself. This may well mean that language teaching will have to be taught more through the curriculum than it has been in the past. In our view this will be wholly a good thing since delivering the curriculum engenders the interest and excitement of learning and language is learned as a result of the need to express ideas about the subjects under study. What we are saying is that it may be more productive for teachers of the deaf to concentrate on delivering a subject on the curriculum rather than taking out a child for 'language work'. Information teaching has been said to be one of the best forms of language teaching! Language work becomes more relevant to the curriculum and we think more stimulating for the child.

One thing that the National Curriculum should very definitely aid is the raising of expectations of what handicapped children can do; and the Government believes, and we agree, that exemptions should be few and far between. However, there is likely to be a significant number of hearing impaired children with handicaps additional to deafness who will be able to reach only the lower levels in subjects. It thus seems likely that staff teaching such children will define more finely graded intermediate steps between target criteria. We see this as a necessary step and still in tune with the spirit of the National Curriculum. Some multiply handicapped children will need levels below level one and here the learning programme is likely to be very individual.

At the other end of the spectrum there is a picture like the one at the grammar school for deaf children where one of us is Principal—here there are currently more than twenty GCSE subjects on offer. And here the introduction of the National Curriculum is likely to *reduce* the choice available to children because it increases the number of subjects a child *must* study and therefore reduces the number of subjects the children may choose. A particularly problematic area is the link between GCSE and A-Level study. For example, because of the constraints of time necessary to pursue the National Curriculum many mainstream schools are no longer teaching three separate sciences but instead following a balanced science course which is the equivalent of two GCSEs. There is now a fear that pupils may find it very difficult to transfer to separate sciences at A-Level. Eventually the A-Level examination must change to bring it in line with the GCSE approach but at the moment we should be very reluctant to change the availability of separate sciences if it reduces the chances of hearing impaired young people pursuing further study in those areas. Certainly students from the Mary Hare Grammar School have a very well established history of achievement in the science and technology area with many now holding high-level positions in industry in these fields. This is clearly an area where the National Curriculum is at odds with the national examination system, a system which hearing impaired youngsters must manipulate if they are to achieve their potential.

It is likely that some hearing impaired children, particularly those with additional handicaps, will be unable to reach more than level one or two in some subjects before they leave school. There is certainly an argument for creating smaller intermediate steps between the target criteria so that some measure of progress can be discerned. Many multiply handicapped hearing impaired children will be working through developmental skills programmes and will require pre-level-one stages if they are to participate fully in the National Curriculum concept. The same must also be true of children with moderate and severe learning difficulties who are not hearing impaired.

Assessment and Testing

The Government has set up the Task Group on Assessment and Testing (TGAT) whose responsibility it is to come up with procedures for testing whether children have reached the attainment targets in various subjects. They have set out to test what children can *actually do* rather than produce measures which merely compare one child's attainments with those of others. This is definitely good news for those with learning problems of one sort or another since its results will emphasise what each child is actually learning rather than setting out to show the mismatch between them and the brightest children in a year group. There are also aims for the testing to give teachers sufficient information to be able to plan for the child's future educational needs.

A variety of methods of testing in addition to conventional written response tests is envisaged by the TGAT. These include computer input, observation of practical procedures and adjustment of a practical outcome or product. Also in the written responses greater emphasis may be placed on multiple choice questions and writing short prescribed responses although it seems unlikely that the TGAT will go the whole way, as has been the case with the GCSE English examination, of basing the testing procedure entirely on coursework. Ministers are already sounding the warning that they do not like 100 per cent coursework options.

An existing problem for deaf children relates to their inability in examinations always to follow the language of examination questions even when they actually know the facts which would enable them to answer the question correctly. In City and Guilds examinations teachers of the deaf have vetted the language of questions and then the paper has been given to both hearing and hearing impaired candidates. In the case of the GCSE, panels of teachers of the deaf have simplified the language of questions (not the questions themselves) and then a special paper has been given to some hearing impaired candidates. It is our view that there is a danger of us ending up with second-class qualifications for deaf children. If the examination board accepts that the simplified language of the question does not simplify the question itself, then they should accept it and give it to all children. Children should be graded on what they know, not on their ability to sort out the sometimes abstruse language used in questions by examiners. This is a difficulty for 16-plus students and we are anxious that it is not repeated in National Curriculum testing on much younger children.

In all aspects of educational assessment greater emphasis is being placed on the child's oral contribution in the classroom and on the ability to respond to visual or tape recorded material. It is vital that testing of such a nature with hearing impaired children is carried on under the direction of, or following the advice of a teacher of the deaf who will be aware of the environmental and practical difficulties of such approaches. A teacher of the deaf should be able to offer advice on how the testing may take place without unreasonably disadvantaging the hearing impaired candidate. As an example of this, a number of profoundly hearing impaired children at the Mary Hare Grammar School for the Deaf who were sitting the GCSE French examination, were required to undertake a listening test, the school being provided with a tape recording by the examination board. When listening, children with such profound deafness need to

be able to make use of visual (lip-reading) clues as well as
what they hear through their hearing aids and of course this is
not available in a tape recording. It was only with some
difficulty that the board could be persuaded to allow us to
bring in a French assistant to actually speak the text of the
tape recording in front of the children. The children all did
very well and we hope that when they go to France they will
speak French to the French face-to-face and not have to do
too much listening through tape recorders!

It is worth pointing out that the use of sign language as an
alternative mode of communication to oral communication is
fully accepted in the National Curriculum—difficult, though,
for a foreign language.

Profiling

The National Curriculum with its attainment targets is part of
an overall aim of the Government that all children should
have carefully documented and presented records of achievement and although the format of such 'profiles' is by no
means finalised the Minister has signalled his intention that
the records should start from the academic year 1990/91.
This, of course, makes it imperative that all schools should
collect, record, and evaluate information on all pupils
immediately.

The major benefits of records of achievement are that each
young person will be able to take a detailed record (and a
summary of it) when they go in search of a job and that when
children change schools a smooth transfer to a new learning
situation can be made. There are many pilot profiling schemes
and one aspect common to most is the contribution made by
the young people themselves. They are given the opportunity
to discuss (negotiate) what goes into the profile and together
with the tutor to set new targets for the next period. The
profiles will include information on non-National Curriculum
areas such as the young person's contribution to the overall
life of the school through extra-curricular activities or service
both in and out of the school.

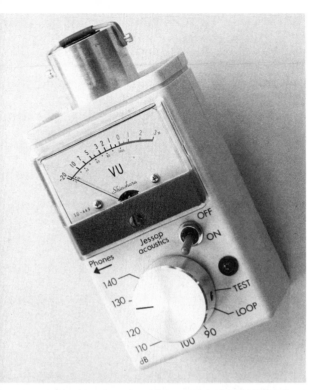

XIII A Jessop Acoustic hand-held hearing aid tester.

XIV *Below:* A Fonix FP30 portable hearing aid test box.

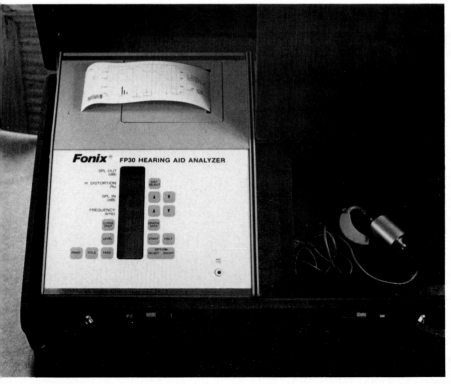

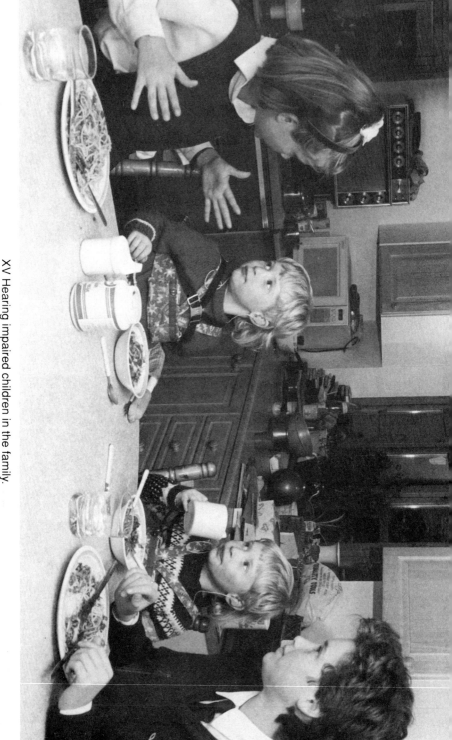

XV Hearing impaired children in the family.

The National Curriculum has been imposed on teachers and children, something which with some people goes against the grain. They feel the education system should be free from the influence of government of whatever political persuasion, but we think it is fair to say that the aims of the National Curriculum to provide a broad, balanced and relevant curriculum would be shared by all teachers. The issue might lie in the definition of those terms. So far it seems that the Government is trying to build on the practice present in the best of our schools and that is good. We just hope that teaching to a National Curriculum will not restrict rather than broaden horizons and that the pressure to teach to pre-defined targets will not stifle the creativity of teachers who teach interesting and exciting things to children who are eager to learn.

Useful Reading on the National Curriculum

PUBLICATIONS FROM THE DEPARTMENT OF EDUCATION AND SCIENCE

The Education Reform Act 1988: The School Curriculum and Assessment, Circular No. 5/89, DES, London, 1989.

The Education Reform Act 1988: Temporary Exceptions from the National Curriculum, Circular No. 15/89, DES, London, 1989.

National Curriculum: Task Group on Assessment and Testing Report. A Digest for Schools, HMSO, 1989.

PUBLICATIONS FROM THE NATIONAL CURRICULUM COUNCIL

Mathematics: Non-Statutory Guidance, York, NCC, 1989.

Science: Non-Statutory Guidance, York, NCC, 1989.

English Key Stage 1: Non-Statutory Guidance, York, NCC, 1989.

Curriculum Guidance 1. A Framework for the Primary Curriculum, York, NCC, 1989.

Curriculum Guidance 2. A Curriculum for All: Special

Educational Needs in the National Curriculum. York, NCC, 1989.

Implementing the National Curriculum—Participation by Pupils with Special Educational Needs, Circular 5, York, NCC, 1989.

7 Listening in Ordinary Classrooms

In Chapter 2 we examined the various types of amplification systems which are available for use with hearing impaired children. For purely practical reasons it is not feasible to use traditional hardwired group hearing aids for hearing impaired children integrated into ordinary classrooms, but apart from this all the other types of aids previously mentioned might be considered. Clearly, personal aids—be they post-aural or bodyworn—will be used by all hearing impaired children, but their limited effectiveness in a busy classroom means that amplification provision must not be limited to these alone. Aspects that need to be considered are how well the pupils hear the teacher, how well they hear their own voices and how well they hear other pupils. It must be appreciated that while modern technology has made a tremendous contribution to the education of hearing impaired children in ordinary classrooms, it cannot yet solve all the problems that arise. For this reason a considerable degree of skill, imagination and flexibility on the part of the teacher is needed if the hearing impaired child is to derive maximum benefit from the education that is being offered.

The main problem facing the pupils with a hearing loss in an ordinary classroom is that of being able to hear what they properly need to hear. Unlike a classroom in a special school, where small numbers of pupils are taught in a small acoustically-treated classroom with a teacher never very far away, an ordinary classroom is often reverberant, filled with children who generate considerable noise, and often the teacher is a considerable distance away. Therefore the three main enemies that affect hearing-aid use—noise, distance from the speaker and reverberation—are all present. These need to be carefully managed on behalf of the hearing-aid user.

The essential requirement is to provide a *good signal-to-noise ratio*. Signal can be defined as the sounds that you want to hear, and noise as any unwanted sound. The signal-to-noise ratio (S/N ratio) is the ratio between the signal level and the level of the noise and is expressed in decibels (dB). A positive S/N ratio, say +15dB, means that the sound-pressure level of the signal is 15dB, higher than that of the noise. A negative value means that the noise level exceeds that of the signal. Whilst it is possible for a normally hearing person to understand speech where the S/N ratio is as low as 0dB, to be able discriminate speech comfortably an S/N ratio of +15 to + 20dB is necessary. However, since it is more difficult to discriminate speech where hearing aids are used, it has been suggested that ideally there should be an S/N ratio of +30dB where this is the case. In an ordinary disciplined classroom where there is likely to be a busy background buzz of 60dB or so, the classroom teacher's voice would have to be raised to a level of 90dB for the benefit of a hearing-aid wearer in order to achieve this, an impossibility for any teacher. The problem is that the teacher is too far away from the child to be able to provide a good signal level at the microphone of the aid. However, by using a microphone reasonably close to the mouth, a radio microphone for example, it should be quite possible to achieve a signal level of 80dB at the diaphragm of the microphone. Indeed, the major reason for providing a radio aid is that it enables a short microphone distance to be used. (Other amplification systems which allow a short microphone distance, such as infra-red systems, would be as effective.) By slightly reducing the level of the background 'buzz', it should now be possible to achieve an S/N ratio of +25dB or even the desired +30dB. Care must however be taken when using radio aids not to have the microphone of the transmitter too close to the mouth, or breath and 'plop' noises will be introduced. Unlike the specially designed microphones which you may see being used very close to the lips by pop singers on TV, the microphones of radio hearing aids are designed to be used between four to eight inches from the mouth. Some research studies have shown that in many ordinary classrooms background noise levels are often considerably above that of a busy 'buzz', and levels as high as 80 to 90dB(SPL) have been found. Where hearing aids are in use, background noise must be controlled for such levels are unacceptable, making even radio hearing aids ineffective.

There are a number of reasons why the S/N ratio needs to be higher when hearing aids are being worn, all mainly associated with their inability to reproduce sound faithfully. One aspect that is important here is harmonic distortion. Harmonic distortion results when a hearing aid itself introduces certain types of sounds which are not present in the original input signal. (It is called 'harmonic' because of the mathematical relationship between the original signal and the additional sounds generated by the aid.) A hearing-aid user may be able to discriminate speech through a hearing aid reasonably well with an S/N ratio of 15dB. He may be able to do equally well in better listening conditions where the harmonic distortion is as high as 15 per cent. Combine the two conditions and the discrimination will plummet! In poor listening conditions the effects of harmonic distortion on speech discrimination are very much greater than would otherwise be the case.

The S/N ratio can be improved by increasing the effective signal level, but greater improvements can often be obtained by controlling noise. How can this be done? There are three main sources of noise: that coming from outside the school site, that arising in the school building and that generated in the classroom itself.

Noise from outside the school site usually originates from road traffic, airports or factories. Noise from such sources needs to be considered carefully when deciding where to site a classroom for hearing impaired children, since controlling such noise is expensive. It is possible to build protecting earth banks, surmounted with special types of fencing, and of course four-inch double glazing helps, unless the windows are open, but the solutions are not easy and would seldom be considered by the appropriate authorities except in very special circumstances.

Noise which arises within the school building may be circulation noise, as children move along corridors, activity noise from playing fields, gymnasia, music rooms, workshops and so on—and noise from ventilation systems and water cisterns. The effects of circulation noise may again be overcome by the careful siting of a classroom within a school if it is to be used as a unit, but for individually integrated children this is not possible. In special schools one would expect the corridors to be acoustically treated; and of course, there are not as many children. Sensible timetabling can help to reduce the effects of activity noise, for example, by planning not to have lessons which demand high levels of concentration and listening when there is a football match outside the window or singing in the hall. Most teachers know when the quiet periods of the day are, and can use this knowledge to the advantage of the deaf child.

Noise generated within the classroom will depend upon the number of bodies within it and the teaching style used. Some classes can be unnecessarily noisy and others commendably quiet. The type of furniture used and the furnishings can make a great deal of difference to the levels of noise, and flooring is of paramount importance. Every classroom with a hearing-aid user within it should have a carpeted floor. This is probably the most important form of acoustic treatment as far as noise control within the classroom is concerned. In some LEAs carpets have been provided specifically for the hearing impaired child, the carpet going with the child when he moves class! Such a solution is clearly more feasible within the primary school than at secondary level.

Reverberation can also be considered to be a form of noise which occurs when the sound signal reflects from walls, windows and other hard surfaces within the room. When this happens the reflected sound reaches the listener having been somewhat delayed by the longer route that it has taken. The delayed sound interferes with the originating signal itself. It might well be difficult to understand a person who is speaking in a very reverberant room or hall. The more the person raises his or her voice, the worse the situation gets. Some large churches used to be notorious for this until the installation of amplification systems overcame the problem.

The time it takes for a sound to stop reflecting is called the 'reverberation time'. More accurately, the reverberation time is the time in seconds needed for a sound to be reduced by 60dB from the instant it stops. It is possible to measure the reverberation time of a room with special instrumentation. It is also possible to calculate it. Typical classrooms have reverberation times which vary from about 1.2 seconds to more than three seconds. By the mid-Fifties it had been shown that such lengthy reverberation times were not suitable for hearing-aid use. It was found that the optimum time for this purpose is not greater than 0.5 seconds. In order to achieve reverberation times of this length, acoustic treatment of the room using sound absorbing materials is necessary. Such treatment should not be confused with treatment for noise generally (although noise and reverberation do of course interact to make matters worse). Different materials absorb different sound frequencies, so it is necessary to use a variety of forms of treatment to achieve the desired end. This is a job for an acoustics engineer; it is not enough simply to lay acoustic tiles on the walls and ceiling. To a normal listener a room with a reverberation time of 0.5 seconds seems rather dead and somewhat unpleasant. Acoustic treatment is expensive so it is not reasonable to expect ordinary classrooms where hearing impaired children are integrated to be so treated, unless a particular classroom is always used for that purpose. It *is* reasonable, however, to expect the classrooms of special units to be treated.

The other main variables which affect hearing-aid use in classrooms are *teaching style* and *types of learning activity*. The most difficult situation for the hearing-aid user is where there is group activity, particularly where this creates considerable discussion and excited chatter. This may be good educationally, but it is very bad acoustically. Accepting that pupils need to talk to each other as they work together, it is in this type of situation that noise levels should be kept as low as possible if the hearing-aid user is to be given a chance. Teachers who attempt to make themselves heard over the din make things even more difficult. Clear, unambiguous

instructions are necessary for hearing impaired pupils, as well
as a check that they really have understood what they have to
do, before the activities start. Group discussion is also
particularly difficult for hearing impaired children. This
situation has to be well managed if it is to be of any benefit to
them. This means that the teacher has to develop techniques
of 'relaying' the contributions of other pupils, both their
questions and their comments. Thus more time is taken up.
However, many teachers have found that the use of such
techniques benefits not only the pupil with a hearing loss but
also many with normal hearing. If the numbers are small
enough, it is possible to make use of a conference microphone
in these circumstances. This is discussed later. Care must be
taken to give the hearing impaired pupil the best chance of
being able to participate fully in the group to which he or she
is assigned. From an acoustic point of view, though not
necessarily an educational one, the easiest situation for the
hearing-aid user is one where the teacher adopts a didactic
approach—talking to a quiet, attentive class! In these
circumstances, particularly if a radio microphone is being used
the hearing impaired child is least disadvantaged compared to
fellow pupils.

It is sometimes a salutary lesson for classroom teachers to
put themselves in the place of their pupils with hearing
impairment. This is easily done by setting up a cassette
recorder where a hearing impaired child normally sits and
recording a morning session. If there is access to any technical
help it is possible for the recording to be made through a
hearing aid similar to the one the child uses and even to do
this using a radio hearing aid for comparison purposes.
Playing the results afterwards in the quiet of one's home, can
be an eye-(or should it be ear?)-opener. By objective, critical
self-appraisal teachers can quickly become aware how their
management of learning in the classroom can make it easier
or more difficult for the hearing impaired child to gain from
the activity taking place.

While radio hearing aids are clearly an absolute necessity in
the ordinary classroom, even where pupils with only moderate

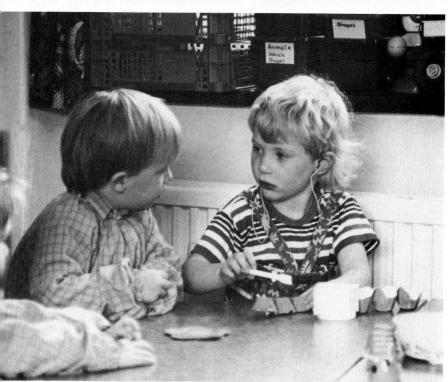

XVI *Above* A) and *below* B): Communication in the nursery.

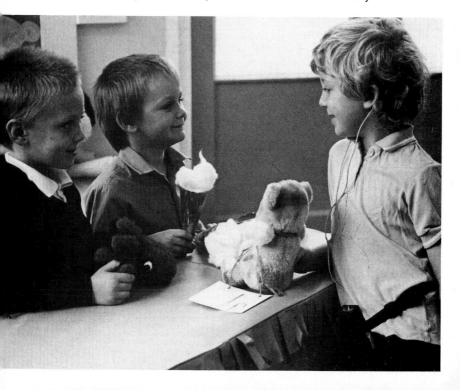

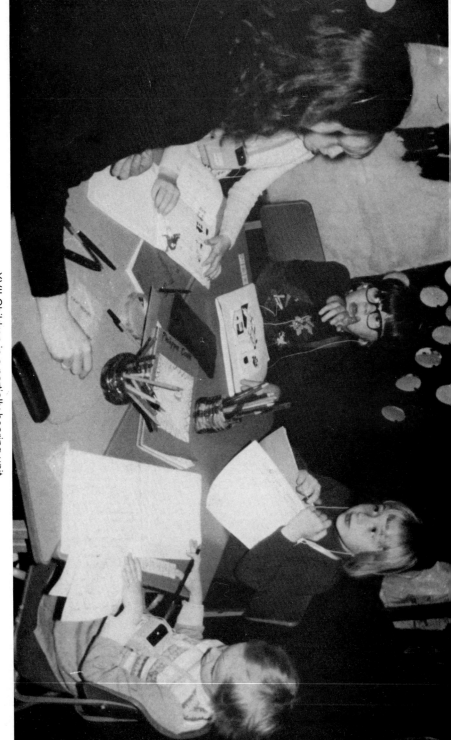

XVII Children in a partially hearing unit

losses are being educated, there is sometimes confusion on the part of teachers about *the use of radio transmitters*—when should they be switched off and when should they be left live? To some extent the answer to this question depends on the age and situation of the child. If the radio system is being used with a toddler in the home, it is probably desirable for the transmitter to be operating for much of the day. A hearing child of similar age will spend much of the time in mother's company as she goes about her work and will overhear most of her conversations with others. For most of the time the mother is happy for this to be the case. In this way the child comes to associate people and events with his immediate surroundings and becomes aware that when people talk, things happen and that language is a powerful tool. The deaf child needs to develop a similar awareness of the power of the spoken word because this will motivate him or her to try to use it. However, a drawback to the use of the radio-aid system is that it does not give the user any clues as to the direction from which a sound is coming. Therefore its continual use with a young child in the home does not allow him the development of sound location skills. For this reason, where conditions are quiet, in a carpeted and furnished lounge for example, there is an advantage in switching over to the child's two personal aids. Because the lounge is quiet and non-reverberant, the signal-to-noise ratio is likely to be as high as when the radio system is in use and the use of two aids will provide some directional information, which in time the child will learn to use.

When the child moves to nursery school or playgroup a more selective use of the radio transmitter is called for. In the home the toddler is part of most things that go on; at playgroup or nursery, this is not the case. Here a number of different activities take place simultaneously and the child is not involved with most of them. The principle here must be that talk transmitted via the radio microphone should have some relevance to the child or the child's activity. It may be addressed to the child as an individual or as part of a group. Teachers therefore need to develop the technique of switching the radio microphone on and off at appropriate moments. Although difficult at first, after a while it becomes almost second nature. Once the child enters primary school this technique should be used from the start. It is important to remember to include the hearing impaired child in larger groups such as assemblies, singing and lunchtime Grace, and for this headteachers and other colleagues should be trained in the use of the transmitter.

It is also the case that in some circumstances it might be desirable for the pupil to switch off the environmental microphone feeding his hearing aid. If noise levels are fairly high, even with the radio transmitter being used, there may be too much noise being picked up by the environmental microphone and this will interfere with the speaker's voice, preventing the reception of a clear signal. Switching off the environmental microphone will improve the signal-to-noise ratio in these circumstances. Clearly, when this is done the user will not be able to hear his or her own voice, so this practice should only be followed when the pupil is not expected to make a spoken contribution to the proceedings.

Although they are more cumbersome and limited in their application, there is a place for the regular use of speech training units with hearing impaired pupils placed in ordinary classrooms, particularly if their hearing loss is profound or severe. Often this will be where the teacher or a classroom assistant has an opportunity to spend a short period of time talking individually to the child in a quiet corner. However, it has been found useful for some children to use a speech trainer for small-group discussions where the microphone can be shared. Infant and nursery teachers have also sometimes found that using the speech trainer with some children is better than a radio aid for quiet story times.

Television, video, radio and cassette recorders occupy an important place in the learning that takes place in modern-day classrooms. It is vital that the hearing impaired child can derive as much benefit as possible from the use of such equipment. Where radio aids are in use, placing the radio transmitter close to the loudspeaker is a common practice, but, while of value, the sound pattern transmitted may be corrupted by mains hum, distortion or rattle. Much better is the solution that takes a direct audio output from the piece of equipment being used to the auxiliary input of the transmitter where it has that facility—and most have. A suitably qualified technician can usually provide the leads necessary to do this. Where speech trainers are used, again there should be no problem in delivering a direct input to these aids, enabling the child to get the best possible sound pattern.

As mentioned above, the use of the *conference microphone* can be very helpful in some situations—the most obvious being small-group discussions. The conference microphone is simply a small, highly directional microphone that can be linked directly either to a pupil's personal aids, a speech training unit, or to a radio receiver in place of a lapel microphone. By pointing it directly at the speaker the user receives a much better signal than from the normal environmental microphone of the aid. The conference microphone helps to reduce the effects of noise and reverberation by providing a better signal-to-noise ratio. Hearing impaired children using this system will find it easier if each speaker in a discussion raises a hand or a finger before starting to speak. The Ewing Foundation publishes a videotape—'Direct Your Remarks at Me!'—about the use of conference microphones with hearing impaired children, which teachers might find helpful.

Occasionally hearing impaired children may wear only one hearing aid, usually a post-aural or possibly an in-the-ear (ITE) aid. Where this is the case, teachers need to be aware of the *head shadow effect*. If the relatively dense mass of the head is placed between a speaker and the microphone of the aid, the signal level of the speaker's voice reaching it will be considerably reduced. This can be as much as 15dB for speech discrimination. In other words the level of speech needs to be 15dB greater when the aid is in the head shadow, for the wearer to be able to discriminate speech as well as when the aid is on the same side of the head as the speaker. This has implications for the seating position of the child in the classroom, and this may need to be changed depending on the particular learning activity that is taking place. The head shadow effect does not apply to a radio-transmitted signal, of course, but it does to the environmental microphone.

Hearing impaired children differ in the amount of *visual information* which they need to support their listening skills. In all but a small minority, audition is the primary route for language-based information, but that is not to deny the important supplementary role of vision in this process. The strategic use of the written word on the blackboard or overhead projector (OHP) and making certain that there are opportunities for lip-reading, both help to ensure that the child makes good use of residual hearing. The use of an OHP is particularly helpful since the pupil can see both what is written and the teacher's face. However, some OHPs have very noisy fans and this noise, particularly when the teacher is using a radio aid close to the OHP, may noticeably interfere with what is being said. It is possible to obtain OHPs that do not need fans and these are much to be preferred.

Positioning the pupil in the classroom needs careful consideration. Before the advent of radio aids it was usual for hearing pupils to be seated at the front of the class so that they were closer to the teacher. The disadvantage of this is that it is more difficult to see other pupils in the class and hear what they have to say. Where radio aids are available it is better for the pupil to sit to one side of the class about halfway from the front. Since the radio signal is equally strong throughout the room, in this position the pupil can hear the teacher as well as anyone else in the class and is able to monitor the contributions of other class members more easily. Lighting is important and the hearing impaired child should sit as close to the window as possible. Many modern classrooms are arranged so that the windows are at the side of the class, so the most favourable position is likely to be halfway back by the window.

School trips and visits away from the classroom are another feature of modern education. One of the points that needs to be considered when planning such trips is how to ensure that the hearing impaired child has the opportunity to use his or her hearing most effectively. The use of a radio hearing aid is an obvious example. If possible, a prior visit by the teacher should be undertaken. This will allow the teacher both to brief some of the people the children will meet and to introduce them to the radio transmitter, which most will be willing to use. It is also useful to be able to identify in advance quiet gathering places where the teacher and others can talk to the children without having to compete with noise and reverberation. Of course the radio microphone also has its uses during breaks and playtimes when children are in the playground or some distance away 'on the field'. The transmitter should have a range of about 100 yards, so this property can be used to good effect. Adults supervising children need to be shown how to use the transmitter and when to switch it on and off. Many a staffroom secret has been 'leaked' by teachers talking privately in the playground in the presence of a live radio microphone!

To be able to use the *telephone* is a necessity in today's world. There are a number of ways that deaf people can communicate on the telephone. For those who have not had the opportunity to develop their listening skills, devices that send written text can be used. The disadvantage of this, of course, is that both sender and receiver have to have such a device fitted (although there are 'relay' schemes whereby written text is sent to a central exchange, from where an operator relays a message to a hearing person by voice, and types back the reply). Fax machines and microcomputers may also be used to exchange written messages. But it is, of course, much more convenient, and indeed opens up many more opportunities for deaf people if they can use spoken communication on the telephone. For those with moderate losses, an amplifying handset may be all that is needed. They may prefer to use this in conjunction with their hearing aid, though some people like to use it direct. For those with a more severe loss, a special inductance loop amplifier fitted onto the earphone of the handset, and used in conjunction with the telecoil position on their personal aids, may well prove satisfactory. Few with a profound loss can use this device successfully, but there is a variant which does work well. This is an amplifier which fits onto the telephone earpiece and sends the signal into the direct audio input of the hearing aid. However, the best solution—though one which is yet to be approved for use by British Telecom—is to use .a direct coupling lead which connects a personal aid, via its direct input, straight into the telephone line. This has been developed at the Mary Hare Grammar School for use by pupils there, and a number of children with losses in excess of 100dB(HL) and many with losses of 95dB to 100dB are able to hold satisfactory spoken conversations over the telephone. However, this is a skill which improves with practice so it is possible that once the device becomes widely available, the great majority of children with a severe hearing loss, and a substantial proportion of those with a profound loss, will be able to learn to use the telephone in the ordinary way if trained to do so. In the opinion of the authors such training should form part of the wider curriculum for hearing impaired pupils, particularly at secondary level. Teachers will need to make special arrangements to ensure that such opportunities for training are provided. There is also a range of strategies which can be learned to help minimise difficulties in understanding that might arise.

Whatever changes will come about as a result of government and local education authority policies, and whatever changes in resourcing there may be, it is clear that the trend, which has developed over the past decade, for a greater proportion of severely and profoundly hearing impaired children to be educated alongside children with normal hearing will continue. This is because it has been shown that where integration policies are put into practice with sufficient attention to resourcing and to the detail of implementation, the results are very encouraging. Hearing impaired children so placed are generally more successful in acquiring a proficient use of spoken English than their counterparts attending most special schools—they have much to learn from the everyday language used all around them by their hearing peers; educational attainments in the formal sense tend to be higher;

they can also live at home and have greater opportunity to make friends with children in their own neighbourhood. For these reasons parents prefer such placement. It is important to appreciate, though, that it is not necessarily suitable for every child, and also that it may be appropriate for some children at the primary stage but not at secondary. But integration can only be successful if very careful and detailed attention is given to ensuring that the hearing impaired pupil has the very best of opportunities to hear and to listen, and of course that what he hears is worth listening to.

8 The Child with Handicaps Additional to Deafness

There is little hard information about the prevalence of additional handicaps in hearing impaired children and there is little doubt that certain additional handicaps, such as Usher's syndrome (where pigmentation of the retina causes increasing visual handicap in addition to the deafness) are often diagnosed very late. Interested readers should see the book by Tucker and Nolan[1] which discusses much of the recent research in this area. There seems to be a tendency to focus on the most obvious handicap and then not to investigate carefully for additional problems. Multi-disciplinary investigation is very important and both parents and teachers should insist on this taking place. Continuing with the example of visual problems and deafness, a hearing impaired child is many times more likely than a normally hearing child to suffer from conditions which cause visual deterioration and yet we know of many children who were never followed up visually when their deafness was diagnosed.

CAUSES OF DEAFNESS WITH ADDITIONAL HANDICAP

Hereditary Factors
It has been reported that there are as many as fifty different genetic syndromes which have a known association with deafness. Obviously most of these are extremely rare conditions. Nance[2] has reported that:

1 Approximately 84 per cent of all genetic cases are transmitted as a recessive trait. This means that both mother and father must be carrying the same recessive gene for that particular handicap.
2 Approximately 14 per cent of genetic cases are transmitted

as a dominant trait. This means that one line of the family carries the gene and that the disability will likely have been seen within that family through the generations.

3 Approximately two per cent of genetic cases are transmitted by a gene on the X chromosome. In this case the males are affected and the females are usually normal.

Additional/multiple handicaps are least likely in hereditary deafness (Vernon[3] puts the percentage at 6.5), though their hearing loss tends to be in the most severe category.

Pre-natal and Peri-natal Factors

The major pre-natal cause of deafness is *maternal rubella* (German measles) in pregnancy. Towards the end of sixteen weeks of pregnancy the evidence would suggest that only hearing will be affected but there is a sharp contrast between the first and the third month of pregnancy. In the first month there could be as many as 50 per cent of the foetuses with major defects, whereas in the third month only about seven per cent. An analysis of all the relevant literature on this area has shown that after rubella in the first eight weeks of pregnancy the chance of having a normal infant is only 35.8 per cent (Sallomi[4]). There is now some evidence that therapeutic abortions are eliminating some of those children who might well have been born with multiple disabilities. Even so, Taylor reported that 30 per cent of his overall population had been deafened by rubella. A vigorous vaccination programme hopes to eradicate rubella altogether but if this is to happen the take-up by teenage girls needs to be close to 100 per cent, and there is no evidence, as yet, that this is happening and there are certainly rubella multiply handicapped children requiring education. There is also a risk of deafness and other handicaps from *birth asphyxia* and *prematurity* (very low birth weight).

Post-natal Factors

Meningitis is the leading post-natal cause of deafness. It begins as an infection of the membranes which surround the brain. Tuberculous (non-suppurative) meningitis is now much less prevalent with better socio-economic conditions and a widespread vaccination programme. Also the highly toxic medicines such as the 'Mycin' drugs, which caused deafness on their own account, have been replaced by less toxic alternatives.

Many forms of meningitis—for example, meningococcal, streptococcal or staphylococci, pneumococcal—were almost always fatal but modern drug therapy has reduced this to about 20 per cent. The illness is very serious and in addition to deafness can result in hydrocephalus, monoplegia, cortical blindness, hemiplegia, mental retardation, convulsions aphasia, brain damage, paralysis and learning disorders. Children severely affected by additional handicap will almost always need a great deal of specialist support and teaching and probably require special school education.

Deafness and Mental Handicap
Many researchers have shown that the incidence of deafness in mentally handicapped people is higher than in the ordinary population. This is true in many types of mental handicap but is particularly so in Down's syndrome where the child has a tendency to increased upper respiratory tract infection, an abnormally shaped skull and very small ear canals. There is also evidence of a progressive high-frequency hearing loss, possibly as a result of premature ageing.

*   *   *

This sketchy coverage of some of the major causes of handicaps additional to deafness serves to highlight the possibility of hearing impaired children suffering mental, physical and further sensory handicap in addition to the hearing problem. Quite clearly such children require varying levels of support since the additional handicap may in itself be a small problem; but it could add the most severe physical and neurological handicap which would make all learning a great feat for the child. The former children may require little extra help but the latter, who may be deaf/blind and/or physically and mentally handicapped, will almost certainly require full-time special educational treatment in a school specialising in the education of multiply handicapped children. In the past such children would probably not have been educated at all but would have been placed in long-term hospital care; but now there are several special schools catering for multiply handicapped deaf children. These schools have in common high teacher : pupil ratios and a need for very high levels of care.

THE DEAF CHILD WITH VISUAL HANDICAP

The main cause of additional sensory handicap in hearing impaired children is rubella, having occurred early in the mother's pregnancy. Others are retrolental fibroplasia, Usher's syndrome (retinitis pigmentosa), meningitis and various unusual genetic syndromes. It is estimated that there are several hundred such children in the country although no official statistics are available. There is evidence that under pressure from SENSE, the National Deaf-Blind and Rubella Association, the government is beginning to take more notice of the problems of this special group. They are beginning to provide some funding in an area where most of what was done was paid for by charitable donation. For many years there has been available the deaf-blind unit, Pathways, which is part of Condover Hall School for Blind Children with Additional Disabilities, Shrewsbury; but now special schools for hearing impaired children—some run by local education authorities, and some in the non-maintained sector (where the school does not belong to the LEA, but the LEA funds individual children to attend the school)—are taking an interest. The Royal School for Deaf Children at Margate has set up a special unit catering for the special educational needs of such children, and others include Elmete Hall School, Leeds; Thorn Park School, Bradford; Royal West of England School, Exeter; and Northern Counties School for the Deaf, Newcastle. One big problem is teaching staff having sufficient training to carry out the work. Currently, training is geared to unisensory teaching not the multi-sensory approach required for deaf/blind children. At least one of the staff at Margate has been trained in both approaches, and this means two years' study additional to that required to become an ordinary teacher. All other staff involved with such children are given in-service training to increase their understanding. We believe that lack of an all-round knowledge can mean that one of the senses, usually the hearing sense, can be neglected. We have seen children with multi-sensory impairment who have useful residual hearing being deprived of the use of that sense because they have not been fitted with aids or they have been fitted ineffectively. It is our view that these children almost always have useful hearing and that hearing aids can at least improve general awareness, reduce behaviour problems and increase their ability to receive other sensory input. At most it can provide the child with an opportunity to learn spoken language through their hearing, a goal which must be fairly high on anyone's list of priorities.

It is our view that the reluctance of some multi-sensorily deprived (MSD) children to wear hearing aids results from the often very late fitting of such devices. All audiologists will recall the increased difficulty of fitting the eighteen- to thirty-month infant as opposed to the six- to twelve-month child. Many professionals argue that the ability levels of multi-sensorily impaired children are underestimated. Clearly, formal intelligence tests cannot reliably be verbally presented to hearing impaired children or visually to blind children. For MSD children it is often only possible to build up a picture of their abilities over a period of time, and using parts of a variety of formal tests. Then, of course, the norms for these tests cannot be used, though a picture can be built up of the child's current level of functioning. From this an attempt can be made to prepare a programme of teaching. Quite clearly, testing of such children is heavily dependent on the co-operation and skill of a variety of professionals, including the audiologist, ophthalmologist, psychologist, parent and teacher. Much of the real information about such children comes from careful observation and one writer reported a boy who had been tested and recorded variously as 'totally blind', 'light perception only' or 'mobility vision' depending on who had tested him, when and where. His mother, however, reported that he could locate a cookie on a table at three feet. She turned out to be correct and her keen observations provided the child's teachers with a starting-point for their educational programme.

At the Royal School for Deaf Children at Margate about one third of the 155 children are multiply handicapped, with 35 being deaf with significant visual handicap. Special units have been developed within the school but the deaf/visually impaired children may be found in all departments of the school since they are placed according to the totality of their needs rather than using the label of a particular disability. Clearly, careful assessment by the school's resident psychologist and specialist teacher of the deaf/visually impaired is very important. On the basis of this assessment the children are provided with the sort of environment they require in terms of lighting, seating and specialised equipment such as low-vision aids. Together with this asssessment and the input of other teachers and carers, a teaching programme is gradually built up. Care for such children must be a whole-school approach since common dangers are a much bigger problem with children whose vision *and* hearing is deficient. Steps, trailing wires, curbs, slopes, walls and moving vehicles on the site can all be serious hazards.

If the child requires a supplementary curriculum including braille, mobility, living skills and the use of low-vision aids they are usually working to individual timetables with very high levels of staff support. In 1982 Bond[6] was involved in the setting up of the department within the Margate school and has highlighted some of the areas which are essential for the best management with such children and others with severe handicaps additional to deafness:

1 Small units are important, with *all* staff sharing ideas on management and involved in the teaching strategies and follow-on assessment and re-evaluation methods.

2 Adequate staffing ratios are important, with one member of staff to two children not unusual.

3 Regular staff meetings which emphasise the learning role for all. These sessions can also act as in-service training sessions.

4 The unit must be well equipped and educational material may need to be designed and made specially for one child according to needs. Appropriate well-made equipment at particular stages in the development of   children with multiple handicaps is crucial.

5 A curriculum consisting of carefully-structured developmental activities and experiences closely linked to skills, which have been analysed and organised in such a way as to make it possible for children and their teachers to achieve realistic goals.

6 Improved liaison between home and school. The school might have a parents' flat, offer parents guidance and training and always be open for parent-school interchange of ideas.

7 An attitude within the department which sets out as a 'problem-solving environment', always willing to try alternative strategies for encouraging learning in the child.

Nationally the pioneering charity SENSE (The National Deaf-Blind and Rubella Association) has done a great deal to persuade government and local education authorities of the need to make provision for such children. The first guidelines on deaf/blind education were published in 1989 by the Department of Education and Science. These guidelines recommend that assessment of educational requirements for the deaf/blind child should begin immediately following diagnosis, and certainly before two years. It is also suggested that LEAs should consider the provision of family support services. Here again SENSE has been a leader in providing a Family Advisory Service (see Appendix). The Department of Education and Science estimates that there are at least eight hundred deaf/blind children of school age of whom only about ninety are receiving education in a specialist deaf/blind unit. While special educational needs should be assessed on an individual-child basis it seems to us likely that more units are required. It is our understanding that a further unit is planned within the Royal School for the Deaf in Manchester. The campaigning of SENSE was influential in the setting up of the first full-time teacher-training course for this speciality at Birmingham University. It is possible that in the future some such qualification may become mandatory.

DEAF CHILDREN WITH SEVERE DISORDERS OF LEARNING AND BEHAVIOUR

As with visual handicap, certain special schools for hearing impaired children are now aiming to provide educational programmes for children with severe learning and/or behavioural, including emotional, handicap. As an example, the Royal School for Deaf Children at Margate has developed facilities which it believes are flexible enough to cater for pupils who have additional impairments which may include:

1 Specific learning difficulties which affect learning, communication and behaviour.
2 A wide range of exogenous handicaps created by, for example, late diagnosis and compounded by other factors such as inappropriate management, placement, expectations or communication, bilingual backgrounds, family disruption, and so on.
3 Behavioural and management difficulties.
4 Physical, physiological, sensory, intellectual impairments including: visual impairment, mental/intellectual impairment; motor and physical handicaps (but not non-ambulant); special dietary problems or needs (e.g., coeliac, hyperkinetic/hyperactive, etc.).

The Royal School for Deaf Children in Manchester now caters only for children with additional handicaps as above and has become the first school for deaf children, to our knowledge, which operates 52 weeks a year. Clearly provision for such children, which often requires one-to-one attention, is very costly indeed and some schools negotiate with education authorities on an individual-need basis.

It is certainly very difficult to group such children in order to cater for their educational needs. Bond[6] suggests that some of the most difficult to sort out are those who on initial examination appear to have no additional major physical intellectual or sensory handicap, but do not develop normally. He has suggested the following possible specific disabilities which alone or in combination seriously affect development:

1 Disorders of short-term memory.
2 Visual attention span.
3 Visual/motor sequencing.
4 Visual spatial planning and organisation.
5 Visual motor learning and visual perceptual skills.
6 Difficulties in simple imitation (for example, of gesture), both gross and fine.

He has also suggested that such children frequently have difficulties in temporal encoding and decoding (e.g., in speech-reading and fingerspelling) and appear to require a higher than usual degree of structure in their learning environment, with plenty of opportunity for success. Bond has also added more factors which may apply to these children:

1 Attention seeking or demanding, and poor on-task and attention-to-task behaviours.
2 Distractibility and impulsivity.
3 Difficulties in interpersonal relationships.
4 Failure in aural/oral approaches.
5 Underachievement in language and reading.
6 Educational records which contain a minimum of medical, aetiological, audiological and psychological information.
7 Involuntary motor behaviours.
8 Muscular rigidity/tension.
9. Clumsiness.

10 Anxiety about failure in reading, maths, written work, etc.
11 Function in verbal educational learning and communication at a much lower level than practical skills and abilities.
12 Occasional flashes of 'brilliance' at a much higher level than the child's assumed level of ability.

But even though the disability is clearly seen, the methodology for teaching the multiply handicapped child may not be readily apparent. There is undoubtedly a need for further research into teaching methodologies. The teaching has drawn much from the methods of teaching the normally hearing but intellectually impaired child. The fact that learning is often very slow and depends on an achievement of one stage before another is attempted has led educationalists to put forward objectives-based curricula where it is necessary to define in great detail what the teaching objectives are, then to assess current pupil performance, implement teaching procedures and then follow up with an evaluation of the effectiveness (outcomes) of the teaching, i.e. a step-by-step painstaking process which is much more 'fine grain' than would be done with ordinary children—even in these days of attainment targets! Techniques of behaviour analysis and behaviour and/or environmental management have been widely used with intellectually impaired children and are now being incorporated in the programmes of some multiply handicapped hearing impaired children. This is in contrast to the method of providing a 'rich' environment, adopted for ordinary children. Clearly, researchers and psychologists need to define how far teaching procedures can be based on the 'enrichment' methods and how much needs to be done using 'task analysis' techniques, where the skills and experiences are identified, ordered into a hierarchy of difficulty, subdivided if necessary, taught, tested and then the effectiveness of the teaching assessed.

The work in this field is extremely demanding both intellectually and professionally, requires great skill and dedication and may be one of the most challenging areas of teaching in which to be involved.

References
1 Tucker, I. G. and Nolan, M. *Educational Audiology*, Croom Helm, London, 1984.
2 Nance, W. E. 'Studies of Hereditary Deafness: Present, Past and Future', monograph, *Volta Review*, 78, (1976), pp. 6-11.
3 Vernon, M. (1969), 'Multiply Handicapped Deaf Children: Medical Educational and Psychological Considerations', Research Monograph, Council for Exceptional Children, Washington DC.
4 Sallomi, S. J., 'Rubella in Pregnancy: A Review of Prospective Studies from the Literature, *Obstetrics and Gynecology*, 27 (1966), p. 252.
5 Taylor, I. G., 'Medicine and Education', *J. Brit. Assn Teachers of the Deaf*, 5 (5) (1981), pp. 134-43.
6 Bond, D. E., 'Management of hearing impaired children who have additional learning and behavioural difficulties', Report on the Proceedings of the Conference of Heads of Schools and Services for Hearing Impaired Children, University of Manchester, Manchester, 1982.

Appendix

Useful Addresses

VOLUNTARY AND PROFESSIONAL ORGANISATIONS
ASSOCIATED WITH HEARING IMPAIRMENT

Breakthrough Trust
Charles W. Gillet Centre, Selly Oak College, Birmingham
B29 6LE. National Director: David Hyslop.
Among other activities, Breakthrough organises family holidays.

British Association of the Hard of Hearing
7/11 Armstrong Road, London W3 7JL.
Work with hearing impaired adults.

British Association of Teachers of the Deaf
Service for the Hearing Impaired, Icknield High School,
Riddy Lane, Luton, Beds LU3 2AH.

British Deaf Association
38 Victoria Place, Carlisle CA1 1EU.
*Hearing impaired adults, including school leavers. Particular interest in
the non-oral deaf.*

City-Lit Centre for the Deaf
Keeley House, Keeley Street, Holborn, London WC2B 4BA.
Further education for deaf students.

College of Speech Therapists
6 Lechmere Road, London NW2 5BU.

Commonwealth Society for the Deaf
Dilke House, Malet Street, London WC1E 7JA.
Aid for deaf children in the Commonwealth.

Ewing Foundation
40 Bernard Street, London WC1N 1LG.
*Aims to promote good educational practice among those who work with
hearing impaired children.*

Jewish Deaf Association
Jules J. Newman House, 90–92 Cazenove Road, London N16
6AB.

Link Centre for Deafened People
19 Hartfield Road, Eastbourne, Sussex BN21 2AR.
Deafened adults catered for on short residential courses.

National Aural Group
Arlington Manor, Snelsmore Common, Newbury, Berkshire
RG16 9BQ.
*Help for parents and professionals working with deaf children. Telephone
helpline, summer schools for families and a range of supportive literature.*

**National Children's Bureau, Voluntary Council for
Handicapped Children**
8 Wakley Street, London EC1V 7QE.
Some very useful publications.

National Deaf Children's Society
45 Hereford Road, London W2 5AH.
*Publishes a quarterly magazine called 'Talk', and has 75 regional
associations in England, Wales, Scotland, Northern Ireland, North-
Western Ireland and the Channel Islands. Useful publications, advice
and advocacy, technical information and pressure group activity.*

National Centre for Cued Speech
London House, 68 Upper Richmond Road, Putney, London
SW15 2RP

National Council of Social Workers for the Deaf
St Vincents Centre for the Deaf, Tobago Street, Glasgow
G40.

National Deaf/Blind Helpers League
18 Rainbow Court, Paston Ridings, Peterborough PE4 6UP.

**SENSE—The National Deaf/Blind and Rubella
Association**
311 Gray's Inn Road, London WC1X 8PT.
*Provides support, advice, advocacy, courses and publications to deaf and
blind children and their families. They are also building up a national*

spread of support centres.

The Royal National Institute for the Deaf

105 Gower Street, London, WC1 6AH.
Technical information, library facilities, mailing sheets and other publications. Regional representation. A concentration on adults—developing interest in post-16 education.

The Association for the Catholic Deaf of Great Britain and Ireland

St Joseph's Mission to the Deaf, Henessy House, 104 Denmark Road, Greenhays, Manchester M15 6JS.

The General Synod of the Church of England Council for the Deaf

Church House, Deans Yard, Westminster, London SW1P 3NZ.

Source of detailed information on schools and services for hearing impaired children

Published annually by the National Deaf Children's Society, 45 Hereford Road, London W2 5AH. All the schools and services for hearing impaired children mentioned in this book appear in the NCDS annual list.

MANUFACTURERS OF RADIO HEARING AIDS

Connevans Ltd, 54 Albert Road North, Reigate, Surrey RH2 9YR.

Phonic Ear, c/o P. C. Werth Ltd, Audiology House, 45 Nightingale Lane, London SW12 8SU.

Radio Link, Cubex Hearing Centre, 324 Gray's Inn Road, London, WC1X 8DH.

Jessop Acoustics Ltd, Unit 5, 7 Long Street, London E2 8HN.

Oticon Ltd, Cadzow Industrial Estate, Low Waters Road, Hamilton, Lanarkshire.

Viennatone, Bonochord Hearing Aids Ltd, Saxon House, London Road, Riverhead, Sevenoaks, Kent TN13 2DN.

Infra-Red Hearing Aids, Pure Tone Ltd, 10 Henley Business

Park, Trident Close, Medway City Estate, Rochester, Kent ME2 4ER.

SUPPLIERS OF AUDITORY TRAINING UNITS

Amplivox Ltd, P.O. Box 105, Kidlington, Oxford OX5 LLJ.

Connevans Ltd, 54 Albert Road North, Reigate, Surrey RH2 9YR.

Jessop-Ralph Ltd, Unit 5, 7 Long Street, London E2 8HN.

Kamplex, P. C. Werth Ltd, Audiology House, 45 Nightingale Lane, London SW12 8SU.

SOURCES OF TECHNICAL INFORMATION

Royal National Institute for the Deaf, 105 Gower Street, London WC1E 6AH.

British Radio Corporation, Lea Valley Trading Estate, Angel Road, London N18. *Loop systems.*

NDES Technology Information Centre, 4 Church Road, Edgbaston, Birmingham B15 3TD. *Also operates radio aid loan service.*

RS Components Ltd, Lammas Road, Weldon Industrial Estate, Corby, Northants.

Pure Tone Audiometers

Amplivox Ltd, P.O. Box 105, Kidlington, Oxford OX5 LLJ.

P. C. Werth Ltd, Audiology House, 45 Nightingale Lane, London SW12 7SU.

Medelec Ltd, Manor Way, Old Woking, Surrey.

Graystad (Medical) Ltd, 36 The Mall, Ealing, London W5 3TJ.

Pure Tone Ltd, 10 Henley Business Park, Trident Close, Medway City Estate, Rochester, Kent ME2 4ER.

Sound Level Meters

Castle Associates, Redbourne House, North Street, Scarborough, Yorks YO11 1DE.

P. C. Werth Ltd, Audiology House, 45 Nightingale Lane, London SW12 8SU.

Bruel and Kjaer Labs Ltd, Harrow Weald Lodge, 92 Uxbridge Road, Harrow, Middlesex HA3 6BZ.

MEG Instrumentation, P.O. Box 32, Sharrow Mills, Eccleshall Road, Sheffield S11 8PL.

Acoustic Impedance Bridges

A and M Hearing Aids Ltd, Faraday Road, Crawley, Surrey RH10 2LS.

Graystad (Medical) Ltd, 36 The Mall, Ealing, London W5 3TJ.

Pure Tone Ltd, 10 Henley Business Park, Trident Close, Medway City Estate, Rochester, Kent ME2 4ER.

P. C. Werth Ltd, Audiology House, 45 Nightingale Lane. London SW12 8SU.

Hearing Aid Test Boxes

Fonix, c/o A and M Hearing Aids Ltd, Faraday Road, Crawley, Surrey RH10 2LS.

Phonic Ear, c/o P.C. Werth Ltd, Audiology House, 45 Nightingale Lane, London SW12 8SU.

Bruel and Kjaer Ltd, Harrow Weald Lodge, 92 Uxbridge Road, Harrow, Middlesex HA3 6BZ.

Rastronics (UK) Ltd, First Avenue, Acumen Centre, Poynton, Cheshire SK12 1FJ.

Jessop Ralph Ltd, Unit 5, 7 Long Street, London E2 8HN. *Market 'Surveyor'.*

TV Tuner and Listening Devices

RTVC Ltd, 323 Edgware Road, London W2.

Ancilaid Ltd, 128 Southdown Road, Harpenden, Herts AL5 1BR. *Infra-red.*

Custom-made Clothing to Carry Hearing Aids.

Appliquéed Children's Clothes, Lucy Morill, 1 Rothwell Road Gosforth, Newcastle upon Tyne NE3 1TY.

Miss C. A. Orrell 47 Sherbourne Road, Heaton, Bolton, Lancs BL1 5NN.

In addition the Technological Information Centre of the National Deaf Children's Society in Birmingham provides information on radio aids and an opportunity to try them.

Index

acoustic feedback—*see* hearing aids

additional handicap 168–178

amplification needs 45–47

anoxia—*see* deafness

assessment 105–7, 142–3, 146–53

attainment targets 146–7

auditory approaches to communication 59–63

auditory training units—*see* hearing aids

auxiliary equipment 162–4

batteries—*see* hearing aids

behaviour disorders 175–8

Bi-lingualism 69–70

bodyworn aids—*see* hearing aids

British Sign Language (BSL) 66, 68–9

controls—*see* hearing aids

Cued Speech 63–4, 79

deafness 8–20

  conductive 9–13

    grommets 12

    middle ear problems 10

    otitis media 11

    outer ear problems 10

    wax 10

  sensori-neural 14–20

    anoxia 17

    German measles 16, 169, 171

    hereditary 14–16

    jaundice 18

    meningitis 20, 169–70

    prematurity 17, 169

    rhesus incompatibility 18

    rubella 16, 169, 171

    viral infections 19

  syndromes 15

distortion—*see* harmonic distortion

Down's syndrome 12, 170

ear 1–8

  mechanism 1–7

  structure 1–7

    cochlea 6

    inner ear—*see* cochlea

    middle ear 3

    ossicles 3, 5–6

    outer ear 1, 4–5

Education Act 1981 127–31

Education Act 1988 142–3

education placement 123–41

ear level aids—*see* hearing aids

earmoulds—*see* hearing aids

fault finding—*see* hearing aids

frequency response—*see* hearing aids

fingerspelling 64–5

gain—*see* hearing aids
genetic counselling 15
German measles—*see* deafness
  (sensori-neural)
grommets—*see* deafness
group hearing aids—*see*
  hearing aids

harmonic distortion—*see*
  hearing aids
hearing, normal
  theories of 7–8
hearing aids 20, 24–56
  acoustic feedback 31
  auditory training units
  (ATU)—*see* speech training
    units
  batteries 48–50
  bodyworn aids 32–3
  cochlear implants 21–2, 44
  controls 29–30
  ear level aids 33
  earmoulds 31–2
  fault finding 47–56
  frequency response 28–9
  gain 26–7
  group hearing aids (GHA)
    36–7
  harmonic distortion 54, 55
  inductance loop 41
  infra-red aids 43–4
  ITE aids 33–4
  output 27–8
  post-aural aids—*see* ear level
    aids
  radio aids 37–43
    Type I radio aids 38–9
    Type II radio aids 39–43

signal-to-noise ratio 155–8
speech training units (STU)
  36–7
hereditary deafness—*see*
  deafness

inductance loop—*see* hearing
  aids
infra-red aids—*see* hearing
  aids
integration 124–6, 131–41
ITE aids—*see* hearing aids

jaundice—*see* deafness

learning disorders 170–1,
  175–8
lip-reading 59, 103–5
localisation of sound 3

mainstreaming—*see*
  integration
manual elements in
  communication 63–70
Maternal Reflective method
  61–2, 80, 121
meningitis—*see* deafness

National Curriculum 117,
  142–53
Natural Auralism 62–3, 80,
  117–19
nursery school 85–94

otitis media—*see* deafness
output—*see* hearing aids

Paget Gorman Sign System

partially hearing units 108–12
peripatetic teachers 100–2
play 95
post-aural aids—*see* hearing aids
prematurity—*see* deafness

radio aids—*see* hearing aids
reading 97–100
rhesus incompatibility—*see* deafness
room acoustics 158–9
  noise 158
  reverberation 158–9
rubella—*see* deafness

SAT 143
school
  preparing children for 94–100
  visits 115–17
sign language—*see* British Sign Language
signal-to-noise ratio—*see* hearing aids
Signed English 65
Sign Supported English 65, 79
speech training units—*see* hearing aids
special schools 112–17
statements of special educational needs 127–9
structured oralism 60–1
syndromes—*see* deafness

telephone 165–6
testboxes 52–6
TGAT 143, 150
theories of hearing 7–8
Total Communication 67–8, 119–21

viral infections—*see* deafness
visual disorders 171–5

Warnock Report 126–7
wax—*see* deafness